The Power of CBD and Essential Oils

Connecting the Dots Between Plants, Receptors, and Health

Dada [signature]

Olivier Wenker, MD, DEAA, ABAARM, FAARFM, MBA

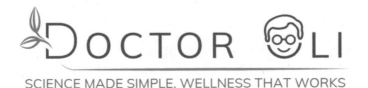

DOCTOR OLI

SCIENCE MADE SIMPLE, WELLNESS THAT WORKS

ISBN# 978-0-9600065-2-6

Printed in the United States of America

Visit doctoroli.com to purchase additional copies.

For information about speaking engagements or to host a book signing, please contact team@doctoroli.com

Edited by Dana Schorr, Ellen Wenker, Lic Phil I, Robert D. Fuller, Ph.D., Richard E. Carlson, Ph.D., Bill Liebich

Table of Contents

Dedication

This book is dedicated to my wife Ellen, my children and their spouses, and a very good and knowledgeable friend, who all watched me blend, mix, measure, heat, cool, and create new products containing different forms of CBD and a variety of essential oils.

Our kitchen often looked like a highly specialized medical laboratory, and sometimes I felt like a mad scientist making sure that the various components dissolved well, had an acceptable or even pleasant taste, could be applied in a user-friendly way, and most importantly, supported healthy body systems, homeostasis, and overall wellness. Each batch fine-tuned the blends to improve absorption and bioavailability rates.

Thank you, Ellen, for your support, and for just shaking your head when seeing me, the nutty professor, in the kitchen with the mess I often made. We gave the expression "shared space" an entirely new meaning.

My Personal Interest in Cannabidiol, AKA CBD

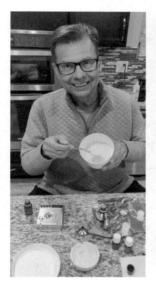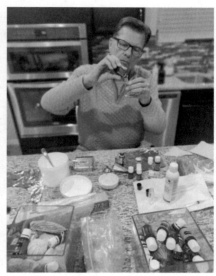

Several years ago, I was diagnosed with a very rare disease called Miller-Fisher Syndrome. This is a subtype of the better-known Guillain-Barré Syndrome, where antibodies start destroying myelin nerve sheaths of mostly peripheral nerves.

With Miller-Fisher Syndrome, this damage is basically isolated to the brain, including the nerves leaving the brain. Both are neurological conditions that cause mild to severe muscle weakness. The damage to the brain and nerves is triggered by an immune system reaction against certain proteins in the tissue that are important for movement, sensation, and function.

The human body confuses the proteins in the brain tissue or nerve sheaths with bacterial or viral proteins, leading to an antibody response with subsequent brain and nerve damage. The typical symptoms of this rare condition are complete ataxia (the loss of full control of bodily movements), eye problems, and lack of deep tendon nerve reflexes.

I was lucky and survived the acute phase of this rare disease. After a couple of weeks in the hospital, I was discharged and went home in a wheelchair. I could barely sit up, and definitely could not stand, without immediately falling to the floor.

I also suffered from eye problems, also called ophthalmoplegia, like double vision, blurred sight, disorientation, and dizziness. The problems can come from damage in the little nerve sheaths of the eye muscles and/or from damage of the eye coordination point in the brain stem.

It was so bad that the neuro-ophthalmologists could not offer any kind of meaningful assistance to enable me to see a single image rather than having blurriness and heavy double vision.

It was then that I decided to make major changes in my life and proactively seek to get my health back. As a first measure, we started to replace highly toxic everyday products such as household cleaners, laundry detergents, soaps, shampoos, toothpaste, and much more with natural, toxin-free, and healthy alternatives. You can read more about this process in my first book (further information found at www.doctoroli.com)

Since I had already exhausted all the treatments offered by modern medicine, like intravenous immunoglobin and plasmapheresis (running my entire blood volume multiple times a day through a special filter to remove any potentially damaging antibodies), I was ready to search for alternative ways to support my brain health.

In addition to using essential oils to support healthy brain function, I also started to search medical literature about other not so common treatment options. I needed to reduce inflammation and further damage to my brain and nerves. I looked at ways to improve my gut function as it is so closely related to proper brain health. I also needed to find out how to support a healthy immune system, since mine had gone haywire during the acute phase of my disease.

Around that time, the U.S. government passed the 2014 Farm Bill, which made cannabidiol (CBD) somewhat legal when used for research. So, I did my own investigations by trying various forms of CBD and then starting to mix them with essential oils. In combination with many other treatment modalities, such as eating healthy ketogenic food, exercising daily, and trying experimental health-supporting activities, I was able to recover extremely quickly from my disastrous condition.

The more I learned about CBD, the more I knew that it was here to stay, at least in my own wellness stash. I had so many positive experiences, and personally did not see any side effects, so it was time to add this compound to my daily regimen. I, and many others in my life, have been consuming CBD ever since.

Throughout this book, I discuss hundreds of scientific research studies regarding different plants and natural substances and their effects on medical conditions. The FDA has classified CBD as a drug, so allowable drug claims are only those approved by the FDA. This book is not a discussion of a few approved *Cannabis*-derived drugs. It represents a review of the current scientific literature on CBD and other compounds obtained from *Cannabis* plants, and therefore summarizes the results obtained by scientists and clinicians.

Some high-quality essential oils have been labelled as dietary supplements. So, when talking about dietary supplements, one can make "structure-function claims", i.e. explain how certain plant ingredients classified as dietary supplements have shown in scientific studies to influence the structure or function of cells in various organ systems.

After reading through literally thousands of references and studies, then stepping back and searching for the big picture, connecting the dots was not an easy task. I hope everyone finds this book informative yet enjoyable.

This book is based on my personal knowledge and experience. It is well known that different people react differently when it comes to natural substances and especially the endocannabinoid system. The information provided in this book is for informational purposes only and is not intended to replace any medical advice or to halt proper medical treatment.

Please consult with your physician and healthcare provider if you have any medical condition, if you take any medication, or if you are pregnant.

After a long medical career using almost exclusively modern, pharmaceutical-based medicine, it has been an eye-opening voyage (re)discovering nature and its treasures like CBD. I am thankful to all who have pointed me in this direction and guided my new education.

Important Note

Today's confusion about hemp and marijuana comes from the use of certain names, especially the word cannabis. While cannabis should be used to describe a plant family, it has been used for over 100 years as a synonym for marijuana. Although CBD and psychoactive THC ultimately come from the same plant species, they are two distinct and different compounds with completely different effects on the human body.

For clarification, in this book, "hemp" will describe the *Cannabis* plant that produces CBD and almost no THC (less than 0.3%). The term "marijuana" will describe the *Cannabis* plant that produces mostly THC (more than 0.3%) with little or non-measurable amounts of CBD. When discussing the botany of the plant, the word *Cannabis* is capitalized and italicized.

If you associate CBD with the word hemp, THC with the word marijuana, and *Cannabis* with the actual plant, you will find it easier to understand this book.

Part 1: History and Background

Lady M. and Her Friend Rasta

The mighty *Cannabis* plant, its individual parts, the products obtained from her, and the laws limiting growth and distribution has been a source of confusion for a long time.

Let's start with confusion number one. What's the taxonomy, or real name, of the plant genus (the biological classification) *Cannabis*? In his original 1753 classification, Karl Linnaeus identified only one species, namely *Cannabis sativa*[1]. But approximately 30 years later, another biologist, Jean-Baptiste Lamarck, started to investigate similar plant material received from India. Lamarck decided to make it a new species with the name *Cannabis indica* (from India).

Currently, *Cannabis indica* mostly originates from India, Pakistan, and Afghanistan, or is cultivated locally. In 1924, the Russian scientist D. E. Janischewsky created yet another new species for the *Cannabis* plant found in Central and Eastern Europe as well as Russia. He called that plant *Cannabis ruderalis*.

The development of modern technology and DNA analysis allowed researchers from the Canberra Institute of Technology to distinguish and categorize almost 200 *Cannabis* plants according to their DNA.[2] They felt that one particular strain should get its own species called "*Rasta.*" Another group of authors suggested to also have a species called *Cannabis afghanica* or *kafiristanica*.[3,4]

Today, it is mostly accepted that we deal with only one species called *Cannabis sativa* and some subspecies (ssp.) called either *ssp. sativa*, *ssp. indica*, or *ssp. ruderalis*. The full name of the *indica* variant would hence be called *Cannabis sativa L. ssp. indica*. The abbreviation L. is used in botany to indicate Linnaeus as the authority for a species' original name.

Another less accurate way to distinguish these subspecies is to look at the mean leaf content of the psychotomimetic (hallucinatory) delta-9-tetrahydrocannabinol, also called THC. If the mean content is above 0.3%, the plant is called *C. sativa ssp. Indica*, and if the mean content is less than 0.3%, it is called *C. sativa ssp. sativa*[5].

C. sativa ssp. ruderalis typically produces mostly the non-hallucinatory cannabidiol, also called CBD. The *rasta* variant produces more THC than other species but has not yet been officially classified in botany.

Nowadays, the species belonging to the genus *Cannabis* are represented by myriads of cultivated varieties. The growers as well as the consumers use non-botanical names to describe the effects or other properties of these variants. Hence, it has been proposed to classify these variants as strains rather than botanical subspecies.[6]

Using 14,031 single-nucleotide polymorphisms (SNPs) genotyped in 81 marijuana and 43 hemp samples, scientists recently showed that marijuana and hemp are significantly differentiated at a genome-wide level, confirming that the distinction between these plants is not only limited to the names of different strains.[7] An SNP is a substitution of a single part of a gene and can potentially change the function the gene. It is the most common type of genetic variation among people, animals, and plants.

The terms hemp, cannabis, and marijuana are used interchangeably but do not describe the same thing. The *Cannabis* plant produces both marijuana and hemp. However, hemp is not marijuana.

As you just learned, *Cannabis* is the genus of the plant. "Marijuana" is used to describe plant material high in THC, while material low in THC (below 0.3%) is called a hemp product. While marijuana is used only for medicinal and recreational purposes, hemp has over 1,000 industrial applications.

If someone wants to get high, they should use marijuana. If they don't want to get high, they should consume hemp.

Take Away Message
- Today it is mostly accepted that we deal with only one species called *Cannabis sativa* and some subspecies (ssp.) called either *ssp. sativa*, *ssp. indica*, or *ssp. ruderalis*.
- *C. sativa ssp. sativa* and *C. sativa ssp. ruderalis* typically produce mostly the non-hallucinatory cannabidiol, also called CBD.
- *C. sativa ssp. indica* is typically rich in THC.
- The terms hemp, cannabis, and marijuana are used interchangeably but do not describe the same thing.
- Hemp has a low or non-detectable amount of THC while marijuana has a high THC content.

History of Hemp and Marijuana

Hemp is one of the earliest known cultivated plants. It originated in Central Asia, and dates back to the Stone Age. In China and modern-day Taiwan, hemp fiber imprints were found in pottery shards over 10,000 years old. Hemp cultivation for fiber production was officially recorded in China as early as 2800 BC and was also practiced in the Mediterranean countries of modern-day Europe early in the Christian era.

The earliest medical description of marijuana appears in the 2nd volume of *Shénnóng BĕnCǎo Jīng,* The Classic of Herbal Medicine, compiled ca. 100 CE from earlier oral knowledge.[8] Earliest archeological evidence of marijuana drug use dates to ca. 600 BCE in Yánghǎi, China. CE is the abbreviation for Common Era and starts with Year One in the first year of the Gregorian calendar. It is the same as AD (Anno Domini) while BCE is short for Before Common Era and is the same as BC (Before Christ).

Around 2,000-800 BCE, the Hindu sacred text *Atharvaveda (Science of Charms)* mentions Bhang (dried *Cannabis* leaves, seeds and stems) as one of the five "Sacred Grasses or Plants" because of its uses in medicine as well as in ritual offerings to Shiva.

A few hundred years later, the *Zoroastrian Zendavesta,* an ancient Persian religious text, refers to Bhang as the "good narcotic.[9]"Just prior to the appearance of Christ, it was reported that the Greeks started using ropes made from hemp fibers and the Chinese invented paper made from hemp.

14

Over the next 100 years, a variety of writers described the use of hemp/marijuana. The Greek historian Herodotus was likely the first to make any mention of *Cannabis* in Western literature when he wrote his description of hemp/marijuana vapor-baths used by the ancient Scythians.[10] Around the same time, Pliny the Elder described in *Natural History, Book 20* that a decoction of the root in water could be used to relieve stiffness in the joints, gout, and related conditions. [11]

Half a century later, Plutarch mentions Thracians using marijuana as an intoxicant. Dioscorides, a physician in Neros' army, listed medical marijuana in his *De Materia Medica*.[12] It's also been speculated that the Ancient Greeks used to burn marijuana to create the smoke for the Oracle of Delphi. [13]

Another Roman physician, Claudius Galen, wrote in *De Alimentorum Facultatibus* that "hemp cakes, if eaten in moderation, produced a feeling of well-being but, taken to excess, they led to intoxication, dehydration and impotence.[14]" When studying ancient literature on *Cannabis*, it seems that at least in the world of the Greek and Romans, hemp was mostly consumed as seeds rather than used as medical treatment.[15]

For the following millennia, hemp and hemp-derived products such as rope and paper started to appear not just in Asian countries but in Europe as well. *Cannabis* started to get more interest in Europe in the 13th century after Marco Polo returned from his journey to the East in 1297 and described in second-hand reports about the wonders of this plant.[16]

Cultivation of hemp then spread throughout Europe during the Middle Ages. It became very important for the Italians who used it for making robust sails for their trading ships and fine clothing. It turned out that canvas sails made of hemp were three times stronger than cotton and were also resistant to saltwater.

This did not go unnoticed by King Henry VIII of England, and he started to impose fines if his farmers did not grow hemp. In 1535, Henry VIII passed an act compelling all landowners to sow 1/4 of an acre with hemp or be fined. During this period, hemp was a major crop and up to the 1920's, 80% of clothing was made from hemp textiles.[17]

It was planted in South America in the 1500s and a century later in North America[18]. In 1616, in the first permanent English settlement in the Americas, Jamestown pioneers began growing hemp to make rope, sails, and clothing. Hemp was so important that just a few years later, the First General Assembly of Virginia created a law requiring farmers to grow hemp.

Hemp quickly became very important for early settlers into the 1800s. Taxes were paid with hemp for over two hundred years, and between the 17th and 18th centuries it was illegal NOT to grow hemp in some areas! The early economy of what is today the United States of America depended on growing hemp.

Some colonies even enforced jail sentences for those who did not participate in what was quickly becoming a patriotic act, especially during the Revolutionary War. In fact, important American historic figures like George Washington, Thomas Jefferson, and Benjamin Franklin were actively involved in the creation of the hemp industry.[19] While both the Constitution and the Declaration of Independence are written on parchment, the rumors have it that some early drafts were written on hemp paper.[20]

So, in 1753, Karl Linnaeus classified *Cannabis sativa* as a plant species. A few years later in 1764, medical marijuana appeared in *The New England Dispensatory*. Hemp was then grown all over America and fields with hemp or marijuana started to appear in Mississippi, Georgia, California, South Carolina, Nebraska, New York, and Kentucky.

In 1850, *Cannabis* was added to *The U.S. Pharmacopoeia* where it is described as a treatment for neuralgia, tetanus, typhus, cholera, rabies, dysentery, alcoholism, opiate addiction, anthrax, leprosy, incontinence, gout, convulsive disorders, tonsillitis, insanity, excessive menstrual bleeding, and uterine bleeding, among others.[21]

In the nineteenth century, when the British physician William B. O'Shaugnessy travelled to India and reported about the therapeutic use of marijuana, the interest towards this plant increased substantially in Europe.[22]

However, things changed suddenly in the United States in the early 1900s. With the creation of The Pure Food and Drug Act, Congress passed a law in 1906 that included marijuana (in addition to alcohol, opium, morphine, cocaine, heroin, and others) to be an addictive drug. That 1906 Act paved the way for the eventual creation of the Food and Drug Administration (FDA).[23]

Just a few years later, during the Mexican Revolution in 1910 to 1920, immigrants fleeing the scene in Mexico brought recreational marijuana with them into the United States. American politicians quickly jumped on the opportunity to promote themselves by labelling hemp and cannabis as "marihuana" in order to give it a bad rep by making it sound more authentically Mexican at a time of extreme prejudice. What was supposed to be a medical or economic discussion became a racist propaganda.

Unfortunately, it worked. Hemp and marijuana were used not just to demonize Mexican immigrants, but also to promote racist agendas against the black population of the time.[24] In addition, certain industries, such as pharmaceuticals and clothing, felt threatened by relatively cheap hemp-derived alternatives. Hemp and marijuana were thrown into the same bucket and all efforts were guided towards prohibiting both.

In 1930, the director of the newly created Federal Bureau of Narcotics realized that he needed more than just opioids and cocaine to establish the importance of the bureau. He decided to add marijuana to the list of substances he needed to regulate, if not eliminate.

Among his alleged quotes are sentences like "There are 100,000 total marijuana smokers in the U.S., and most are Negroes, Hispanics, Filipinos, and entertainers. Their Satanic music, jazz and swing, results from marijuana use. This marijuana causes white women to seek sexual relations with Negroes, entertainers, and any others... The primary reason to outlaw marijuana is its effect on the degenerate races."[25] It was the birth hour of the war against marijuana and any other hemp-derived products.

The director was soon supported by an owner of a huge chain of newspapers, who hated Mexicans because he lost some of his timber land to them. He was also heavily invested in creating paper from his timber enterprise. Cheap hemp paper was not what he wanted. Then, some pharmaceutical giants at the time had trouble standardizing marijuana drugs and did not like the idea that people could just grow them by themselves without having to purchase expensive drugs.

Together, they decided to support a new law, and in 1937 the Marijuana Tax Act was established, under which taxes were imposed on the sale of hemp and marijuana. The Act itself did not criminalize the possession or usage of hemp or marijuana, but it included penalties and enforcement provisions to which marijuana and hemp handlers were subject.[26]

Cannabis including hemp was therefore criminalized for mostly political reasons in the United States in 1937, against the advice of the American Medical Association at that time.[27] The Act was then finally declared unconstitutional in 1969.[28] But soon after, the war on marijuana intensified again and the Comprehensive Drug Abuse and Prevention Control Act, more commonly known as the Controlled Substances Act (CSA), was put into law in 1970 and 1971.

Drugs and other substances that are considered controlled substances under the CSA are divided into five schedules.[29] An updated and complete list of the schedules is published annually in Title 21 Code of Federal Regulations (C.F.R.) §§ 1308.11 through 1308.15.

Substances are placed in their respective schedules based on whether they have a currently accepted medical use in treatment in the United States, their relative abuse potential, and likelihood of causing dependence when abused.

Schedule I Controlled Substances

Substances in this schedule have no currently accepted medical use in the United States, a lack of accepted safety for use under medical supervision, and a high potential for abuse.

Schedule II/IIN Controlled Substances (2/2N)

Substances in this schedule have a high potential for abuse which may lead to severe psychological or physical dependence.

Schedule III/IIIN Controlled Substances (3/3N)

Substances in this schedule have a potential for abuse less than substances in Schedules I or II and abuse may lead to moderate or low physical dependence or high psychological dependence.

Schedule IV Controlled Substances

Substances in this schedule have a low potential for abuse relative to substances in Schedule III.

Schedule V Controlled Substances

Substances in this schedule have a low potential for abuse relative to substances listed in Schedule IV and consist primarily of preparations containing limited quantities of certain narcotics.

Marijuana was put into Schedule I and interestingly, there was no distinction made between marijuana and hemp. It is also worth mentioning that at that time, we already had scientific articles in medical literature describing the long history of medical marijuana and reporting the medical benefits of marijuana on illnesses like seizures. Despite this knowledge at the time, marijuana (and hemp) was classified as having no acceptable medical use.

This Act also required farmers to obtain a special permit allowing them to grow industrial hemp. Because of the issue surrounding the legality, or better illegality, of growing hemp, most hemp products in the past decades have been imported into the United States. The requirement for imports is that hemp products cannot have more than 0.3% THC in them.

In 2014, the President of the United states signed the 2014 Farm Bill under which industrial hemp could be cultivated for research purposes. Since then, sales of hemp-derived CBD have exploded, and so did research on CBD. Effective January 2017, the Drug Enforcement Agency (DEA) created a new controlled substances code number (7350) for marijuana extracts.[30] The DEA ruling was very clear that extracts of "any plant of the genus *Cannabis*, other than the separated resin" are included in Code 7350 in Schedule I of the CSA.[31]

In the summer of 2018, the FDA granted approval for a non-synthetic plant-based CBD drug called Epidiolex for the treatment of seizures associated with two rare and severe forms of epilepsy, Lennox-Gastaut Syndrome and Dravet Syndrome, in patients two years of age and older.

21

The FDA also mentioned that this is the first FDA-approved drug that contains a purified drug substance derived from marijuana. Interestingly, the FDA did not clarify that CBD is from hemp and not from marijuana.

In the same statement, the FDA explained how it prepares and transmits, through the U.S. Department of Health and Human Services, a medical and scientific analysis of substances subject to scheduling, like CBD, and provides recommendations to the Drug Enforcement Administration (DEA) regarding controls under the Controlled Substances Act (CSA). The DEA is required to make a scheduling determination.[32]

The DEA then announced shortly thereafter that drugs including "finished dosage formulations" of CBD with THC of less than 0.1% will be listed in schedule V of the Controlled Substances Act, as long as the medications have been approved by the FDA.[33] Schedule V classifies a drug as having a low potential for abuse.

Three months later, on December 20th, the President of the United States signed the 2018 Farm Bill. Under this bill, CBD has been de-scheduled from its Schedule V status. In other words, within just a few months, CBD went from being a Schedule I to a Schedule V substance and then to an unscheduled substance, at least at the federal level.

The 2018 Farm Bill contained language about hemp and hemp-derived products. Hemp is now legally defined as a *Cannabis* plant or part of the *Cannabis* plant that has a THC concentration of not more than 0.3% on a dry weight basis. Also, in order to be federally legal, the CBD product must be derived from hemp grown by a licensed business with official federal and state government approval.

However, much of today's hemp is grown by companies without these permits, which makes many CBD products illegal independent of where and how they are sold. To make things more complicated, the Farm Bill also allows individual states to make and enforce their own, sometimes more restrictive, laws.

Immediately after the signing of the Farm Bill, the FDA issued a warning statement regarding the use of hemp-derived products.[34] Here is some of it:

> *Statement from the FDA Commissioner Scott Gottlieb, M.D., who served as the 23rd Commissioner of the FDA from May 2017 to April 2019, on signing of the Agriculture Improvement Act and the agency's regulation of products containing cannabis and cannabis-derived compounds.*
>
> "Today, the Agriculture Improvement Act of 2018 was signed into law. Among other things, this new law changes certain federal authorities relating to the production and marketing of hemp, defined as *Cannabis* (*Cannabis sativa L.*), and derivatives of *Cannabis* with extremely low (less than 0.3% on a dry weight basis) concentrations of the psychoactive compound delta-9-tetrahydrocannabinol (THC). These changes include removing hemp from the Controlled

Substances Act, which means that it will no longer be an illegal substance under federal law.

Just as important for the FDA and our commitment to protect and promote the public health is what the law didn't change: Congress explicitly preserved the agency's current authority to regulate products containing *Cannabis* or *Cannabis*-derived compounds under the Federal Food, Drug, and Cosmetic Act (FD&C Act) and section 351 of the Public Health Service Act.

We're aware of the growing public interest in *Cannabis* and *Cannabis*-derived products, including cannabidiol (CBD). This increasing public interest in these products makes it even more important with the passage of this law for the FDA to clarify its regulatory authority over these products. In short, we treat products as we do any other FDA-regulated products — meaning they're subject to the same authorities and requirements as FDA-regulated products containing any other substance. This is true regardless of the source of the substance, including whether the substance is derived from a plant that is classified as hemp under the Agriculture Improvement Act.

In particular, we continue to be concerned at the number of drug claims being made about products not approved by the FDA that claim to contain CBD or other *Cannabis*-derived compounds. Among other things, the FDA requires a

Cannabis product (hemp-derived or otherwise) that is marketed with a claim of therapeutic benefit, or with any other disease claim, to be approved by the FDA for its intended use before it may be introduced into interstate commerce.

Additionally, it's unlawful under the FD&C Act to introduce food containing added CBD or THC into interstate commerce, or to market CBD or THC products as, or in, dietary supplements, regardless of whether the substances are hemp-derived. This is because both CBD and THC are active ingredients in FDA-approved drugs and were the subject of substantial clinical investigations before they were marketed as foods or dietary supplements. Under the FD&C Act, it's illegal to introduce drug ingredients like these into the food supply, or to market them as dietary supplements.

We recognize the potential opportunities that cannabis or cannabis-derived compounds could offer and acknowledge the significant interest in these possibilities. We're committed to pursuing an efficient regulatory framework for allowing product developers that meet the requirements under our authorities to lawfully market these types of products."

Am I the only one who thinks this is somehow backwards? The FDA decides to approve a pharmaceutical version of CBD and now calls the natural ingredients of the hemp plant "drug ingredients." And because CBD is now a drug ingredient, they claim authority over any regulation on whether CBD can be used as food or a dietary supplement. At least they labeled the very nutrient-rich hemp hearts as GRAS (Generally Regarded As Safe) and allow them to be consumed.

It is just another example of the pharmaceutical industry recreating or using nature in a lab and then being protected by the FDA's regulations of the consumption of the natural products, even if those natural products have been used safely for thousands of years. This does make sense in cases where the natural products have shown to have potential to harm people. After all, the FDA was created to protect American consumers.

But when we look at all the scientific evidence on hemp and CBD that has been published over the past few years, there is just nothing substantial about harm to humans. The worst effect described was dizziness in high doses. No one died from CBD or suffered any major negative side effects. In contrary, all reports describe the positive effects that this compound has on the human body. It seems to be so important, that not only do humans have receptors for CBD in various tissues, but we also create our own CBD-like compounds in the body.

I very much hope that the FDA will quickly come to its senses and follow the example set by the House, Senate, and President and remove CBD from their authority, opening it for human consumption without roadblocks and limitations.

I also hope that the FDA takes one more look at the medical evidence concerning THC, because at this time it is still classified as a Schedule I compound with high potential for abuse and no medical benefits whatsoever, but there are medical benefits associated with the use of marijuana. The FDA has been charged with keeping us, the population, safe from bad products and false claims, but I want to see it controlling the purity and quality of CBD products instead of limiting the use.

Interestingly, the FDA is not alone struggling with this issue. According to a recent article, it is a worldwide problem.[35] For example, the European Commission has recently reclassified CBD as "Novel Food" which opens many possibilities for future scenarios under which CBD products can be sold and consumed, namely as food instead of a drug. Most European countries have a zero-tolerance policy for natural or synthetic THC unless it is approved as a drug.

Latin American countries are on the move to legalize both CBD and THC, including the agricultural production of hemp. There is a good business opportunity for some of these countries to become a supplier for this exploding worldwide market. A few years ago, Uruguay legalized both CBD and THC for recreational use. Other countries such as Columbia, Argentina, and Mexico are all catching up with their laws.

Asian countries, including India and the Philippines, introduced laws allowing medical professionals to prescribe *Cannabis* products for certain medical conditions. And Australia only permits CBD to be used as medical drug.

In the United States, we often have the feeling that the freedom of the population is severely impacted by the

27

rules from the FDA. However, as with many other products, we see that the rules and regulations in other parts of the world are even more restrictive. Nevertheless, it is time to release CBD from the iron grip of regulators since it has proven to be safe in every application to date and the results can be spectacular for many conditions.

Federal law, FDA regulations, and state laws are currently in complete chaos. Almost half of the United States has now legalized medicinal marijuana, several states have legalized recreational use, a few completely forbid any form of product coming from the *Cannabis* plant, and others have legalized CBD-only use.[36]

The Farm Bill specifically mentions that the states have the authority to create and enforce their own laws. When we look at today's legal landscape regarding CBD, we find everything from legal to illegal when it comes to sales, personal possession, and consumption of CBD. Various web sites are trying hard to keep up with the constantly changing State laws and keep us updated.

As per early 2019, the following rules were in place:[37,38]

> Legal as defined in 2018 Farm Bill: Alabama, Arizona, Arkansas, Connecticut, Delaware, Florida, Georgia, Hawaii, Illinois, Indiana, Iowa, Kansas, Kentucky, Louisiana, Maryland, Minnesota, Missouri, Montana, New Hampshire, New Jersey, New Mexico, New York, North Carolina, North Dakota, Ohio (CBD has to be sold in licensed dispensaries), Oklahoma, Pennsylvania, Rode Island, South Carolina, Tennessee, Texas, Utah, Virginia, West Virginia,

Wisconsin, and Wyoming. (Remember, legal means that the growers must be approved and licensed by the state in question. Legal does not mean that you can just produce, buy, sell, and/or consume any CBD. Federal and state laws still apply to legal CBD.)

Hemp- and marijuana-derived CBD produced within the state is legal under the state's recreational marijuana laws. Interstate commerce with CBD from non-approved growers is illegal: Alaska, California, Colorado, Maine, Massachusetts, Michigan, Nevada, Oregon, Vermont, and Washington.

CBD is illegal and anyone selling and potentially possessing CBD can be prosecuted: Nebraska, South Dakota, and Idaho.

Disclaimer: Please do not rely on this information because the rules, laws, and regulations constantly change. I cannot guarantee that by the time you are reading this information that it is still valid. Any decision on whether to use CBD in any way, shape, or form is your decision and cannot be based on the information presented in this book as it might be outdated as soon as it has been printed.

In March 2019, it was made public that about a dozen states have a provision in their statutes ordering them to declassify any drug or substance as soon it has been declassified by the federal government. This opens new avenues for the legalization of hemp products, at least in some states. In the coming months and years, we will see many legal changes within the U.S. as well as around the world. It remains to be seen how consumer-friendly these changes will be.

Take Away Message

- Hemp is one of the earliest known cultivated plants.
- *Cannabis* started to get more interest in Europe in the 13th century after Marco Polo returned from his journey to the East.
- The early economy of what is today the United States of America depended on growing hemp.
- With the creation of The Pure Food and Drug Act, Congress passed a law in 1906 that labelled marijuana to be an addictive drug.
- Immigrants fleeing the Mexican Revolution in 1910 to 1920 brought recreational marijuana with them into the United States. American politicians labelled hemp and cannabis as "marihuana" to make it sound more authentically Mexican at a time of extreme prejudice.
- Hemp and marijuana were thrown into the same bucket and all efforts were guided towards prohibiting both.
- In 1937 the Marijuana Tax Act was established, and taxes were imposed on the sale of hemp and marijuana.
- The Controlled Substances Act was put into law in 1970 and 1971.
- There was no distinction made between marijuana and hemp.
- Most hemp products in the past decades have been imported into the United States.
- In 2018, the President of the U.S. signed the Farm Bill, which de-scheduled CBD from its Schedule V status.
- Immediately after the signing of the Farm Bill, the FDA issued a warning statement regarding the use of hemp-derived products.

- The FDA decided to approve a pharmaceutical version of CBD.
- Because CBD is now a drug ingredient, the FDA claims authority over any regulations.
- The European Commission has recently reclassified CBD as "Novel Food."
- Internationally, many countries are on the move to legalize both CBD and THC, while others allow medical professionals to prescribe *Cannabis* products for certain medical conditions.
- Federal law, FDA regulations, and state laws are currently in complete chaos.
- In the coming months and years, we will see many legal changes within the U.S. as well as around the world. It remains to be seen how consumer-friendly these changes will be.

Hemp Plants

Industrially grown hemp is currently used for a variety of products, including health foods (edible seeds), organic body care, clothing, rope, construction materials, paper, canvas, biofuel, plastic composites, caulk, fiberglass, insulation materials, and more.

Hemp needs less water than other crops and very little fertilizer, if at all. The hemp plant is naturally resistant against many pests, and because it grows very dense, it does not allow weeds to disturb the fields. Hence, no pesticides or herbicides are needed, making this an eco-friendly crop. Unfortunately, testing shows that most hemp and marijuana products contain pesticides, herbicides, as well as fertilizer residues.

Hemp also produces as much paper from a one-acre field as two to three acres of trees. As a reminder, hemp can be harvested annually, while trees will take many years or decades to grow. In addition, the quality of hemp paper is superior to tree-based paper. It can last hundreds of years without degrading, can be recycled many more times than tree-based paper, and requires fewer toxic chemicals in the manufacturing process than paper made from trees.[39] Hemp is very environmentally friendly if grown without toxic chemicals. All-in-all, a win-win for the economy and the environment.[40]

Hemp Seeds

Hemp seeds are popular for their high nutrient content and have been an important source of nutrition for thousands of years. Hemp seeds typically contain over

30% oil and up to 35% protein, in addition to considerable amounts of dietary fiber, flavonoids, vitamins, and minerals. After being harvested, these seeds can be whole hulled or shelled or they can be pressed for oil.

In general, hemp seeds intended for ingestion are extremely low in CBD and THC or have none at all. However, researchers discovered that, depending on the extraction method used, the Δ9-THC concentrations in these hemp seeds could be as high as 1,250% of the legal limit.[41]

Hemp seeds are regarded as highly nutritious because of the outstanding nutrients they provide. Whole seeds provide the best nutritional value, since shelled seeds, also known as hemp hearts, are much lower in fiber content. Hemp seeds are rich in proteins, which are made of chains of different types of amino acids. We can classify the 21 human amino acids into three groups: essential, non-essential, and conditional amino acids.[42]

Essential amino acids must be consumed since they cannot be produced by the body, hence the name essential. The nine essential amino acids are histidine, isoleucine, leucine, lysine, methionine, phenylalanine, threonine, tryptophan, and valine.

Non-essential amino acids are produced in our bodies but are still necessary for the body to function. The four non-essential amino acids are alanine, asparagine, aspartic acid, and glutamic acid.

Conditional amino acids are usually not essential, except in times of illness and stress. The eight conditional amino acids are arginine, cysteine, glutamine, tyrosine, glycine, ornithine, proline, and serine.

Proteins from animal sources have mostly complete amino acid profiles, whereas proteins from plant-based compounds contain mostly incomplete amino acid profiles. Hemp seed proteins contain all nine essential amino acids.

The two main proteins in hemp seeds are albumin (~30%) and edestin (~70%). Both proteins are easily digestible and serve as building blocks for hormones, immunoglobulins, hemoglobin (your carrier for oxygen), and enzymes. These proteins have exceptionally high levels of the amino acids arginine and L-tyrosine. Arginine, or L-arginine to be specific, is an amino acid precursor to nitric oxide (NO).[43] Release of NO in the wall of blood vessels results in vasodilatation[44], which means that NO widens blood vessels and therefore increases blood flow.

This effect is important for people with high blood pressure or cardiovascular diseases since arginine has been shown to lower blood pressure, reduce fasting blood sugar and cholesterol, as well as improve lipid profiles thereby reducing cardiovascular risks.[45,46]

The body uses L-tyrosine to produce the neurotransmitters dopamine and noradrenaline. Both compounds are depleted during stress. L-tyrosine supplementation can increase the levels of these important neurotransmitters. As a result, clinicians speculate that it could prevent a decline in cognitive function in response to physical stress.[47]

Hemp seed oil is made of 80% polyunsaturated fatty acids (PUFAs) and is an exceptionally rich source of the essential fatty acids linoleic acid and alpha-linolenic acid. The omega-6 to omega-3 ratio in hemp seed oil is normally between 2:1 and 3:1, which is considered to be optimal for human health.[48]

Hemp also contains healthy flavonoids, like grossamide, which is known for its neuroprotective action.[49] Other plants, like peppers, also contain grossamide. The anti-inflammatory and neuroprotective effects of grossamide result from inhibition of secretion of inflammatory compounds.

Crushed hemp seeds and hemp flour are used to make bread, granola, protein powders, and animal food. Hemp oil is used for biofuels, lubricants, paint, varnish, cosmetics, body care products, salad dressings, margarine, and ink. Hemp stalks are made of two important parts: hurd and bast fibers. Hurds, or shivs, are materials from the white woody inner core and are used for products like insulation materials, mulch, fiberglass, chemical absorbents, and even concrete (hemp-crete).

Bast fibers come from the green outer layer of the hemp stalk. These fibers are long, thin, and strong. They also have antibacterial properties, negating the need for chemicals to preserve the fibers. Bast fibers are used to produce rope, nets, canvas, paper, clothes, shoes, bags, carpets, and bio-composites.

The entire stalk can be used in the production of cardboard, filters, paper products, and as biofuel feedstock. As a natural substitute for cotton and wood fiber, hemp can also be pulped using fewer harsh chemicals because of its low lignin content. Its natural brightness can reduce or eliminate the need for chlorine bleach.

On December 20th, 2018, the FDA released the following wording regarding the legal distribution of hemp seed products intended for ingestion:

> "We are able to advance the lawful marketing of three hemp ingredients today. We are announcing that the agency has completed our evaluation of three Generally Recognized as Safe (GRAS) notices related to hulled hemp seeds, hemp seed protein, and hemp seed oil and that the agency had no questions regarding the company's conclusion that the use of such products as described in the notices is safe.
>
> Therefore, these products can be legally marketed in human foods for these uses without food additive approval, provided they comply with all other requirements and do not make disease treatment claims."[50]

Hemp

Members of the genus *Cannabis*, including hemp and marijuana, typically are either male or female plants. Male plants produce vast amounts of pollen that can spread with the wind over large geographical areas and pollinate female plants. If male and female flowers are produced by individual male or female plants respectively, the plant is called dioecious.[51] If however the same individual plant has both male and female flowers, the plant is called monoecious.[52] Plants containing male and female flowers are also called hermaphrodites or in short "Hermis."

Commercially grown hemp is from fields containing both male and female plants. Both sexes have different characteristics which enable growers to tell them apart. Male plants and pollinated female plants are both low in cannabinoids. Male plants form pollen sacks from which they release pollen. Female plants form sexual organs intended to be pollinated. Such sexual organs are called pistils and they grow inside the flower. Early in the plant lifecycle the pistils will look like white hair. As the female plant matures, these white pistils turn orange and red, indicating that the plant is ready to be harvested.

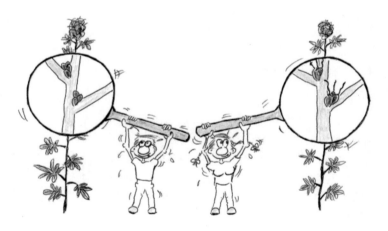

Difference between male and female Cannabis plants
(Pollen sacks versus pistils)

Male plants typically die off after they are done pollinating, and it is the female plants that grow to full maturity. Once fertilized or pollinated, female plants spend most of their energy on producing seeds instead of THC. This is where we get hemp seeds from.

When male plants are missing, female plants don't get pollinated and get, sexually speaking, frustrated. In this frustration, they increase the efforts to attract pollen by enhancing the production of a resin-like substance. Pollen sticks easily to this gluey substance. The longer it takes for the female to get pollinated, the more frustrated she gets, and the more resin-like substance will be excreted.

As a result, female flowers will be coated with cannabinoid-rich resin. So, a properly pollinated female *Cannabis* plant will concentrate its entire energy to produce offspring, AKA hemp seeds. A non-pollinated female *Cannabis* plant will concentrate its entire energy to try to get pollen to stick (to be pollinated) by producing THC-containing resin.

The resin is excreted from structures called trichomes.[53] In hemp and marijuana plants they are translucent, mushroom-like structures mostly growing within the flowers and on the leaves of a female plant. These trichomes are tiny manufacturing facilities and produce THC-rich resin, CBD, other cannabinoids, as well as terpenes.

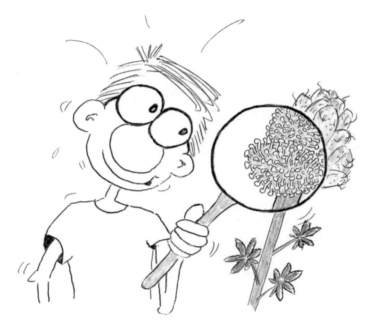

Resin-producing trichomes

Terpenes are an oily substance with a particular taste and aroma. You might remember that essential oils also contain terpenes. In fact, thousands of compounds belonging to the family of terpenes have been identified in essential oils.[54] Essential oils mainly have two distinct groups of chemical compounds. First, hydrocarbons made up almost exclusively of terpenes (monoterpenes, sesquiterpenes, and diterpenes), and second, oxygenated terpenes which are mainly esters, aldehydes, ketones, alcohols, phenols, and oxides.

The terpenes in the various marijuana strains are what gives them their unique taste and aroma profiles. The aroma differences among strains are substantial,[55] and we will see later in the book that they have an important function.

Cannabis plants (hemp and marijuana) have roots, stems or stalks, leaves such as fan leaves and sugar leaves, colas (which is where the flowers or buds grow), pistils, trichomes, and calyxes which are the actual flowers of the plant. Roots and stalks are mostly used for industrial products. Fan leaves are the typical *Cannabis* leaves and used globally in logos to represent marijuana. They fan out nicely and grow from the nodes on the stalk.

Male plants have sturdier stalks, and their fan leaves are not as large and rich as those from female plants. Sugar leaves are very small leaves found in the flower. They are sprinkled with trichomes giving them a white sugary appearance.

Fan leaves have significantly fewer trichomes compared to sugar leaves. Therefore, more cannabinoids and terpenes are produced in the flower compared to other parts such as the fan leaves. A cola can represent an entire cluster of buds. The highest (from the ground) cola on a *Cannabis* plant is sometimes called the main cola.

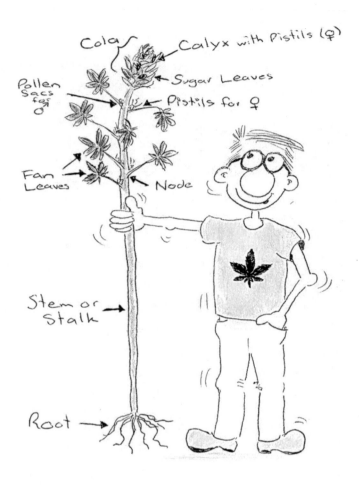

Anatomy of a Cannabis plant

Growing Hemp

The *Cannabis* plant grows in two stages: the vegetative stage and the flowering stage. It is difficult to distinguish between male and female plants during the vegetative stage, which is the first six to eight weeks of growth.

41

After that, the differences between the two sexes start to show, like pre-flowers on female plants.

Also, males will have pollination sacks without hair along the stem where their leaves branch off, compared to similar structures with pistils on female plants. Male plants have sturdier and typically shorter stalks, and female plants will have fuller and more densely distributed fan leaves. In maturing plants, large and full flower buds appear on females, compared to small sparsely populated bud-like structures showing on males.

It takes longer to distinguish male from female plants in outdoor fields compared to indoor cultivation. Exposure to long periods of sunlight in the summer on the fields slows down the flowering stage. This is why indoor cultivators use a specific time schedule to control the amount of light a plant receives.

However, in the vegetative stage the plant needs light in order to grow. In nature, the shorter days and longer nights of the fall and winter seasons cause the *Cannabis* plant to start flowering before it is too late and the lifecycle of the plant ends. Once the plant enters the flowering stage, distinct male and female differences start to show.

Hermis, or two-gendered plants, as well as male plants, are typically not desired by marijuana growers as such plants do pollinate females resulting in more hemp seeds and less THC production. Marijuana growers will therefore periodically check their crop and remove unwanted plants in order to produce female-only colonies with high THC and low CBD yield.

Hybridization is the merging of differing gene pools to create unique offspring. Extensive cultivation of marijuana plants led to the creation of numerous fertile hybrids that can maintain their characteristics over different generations. This cross-hybridization is the reason we have hundreds of different strains of this plant.

Cannabis Leaf Fingers?

The typical marijuana logo mostly shows seven "fingers" on the leaf. I have been asked many times whether the fact that a marijuana leaf has five or seven fingers indicates if the plant has grown outside in nature or inside under controlled conditions. The number of fingers on a leaf depends on a variety of factors.

First, different subspecies of *Cannabis* have different leaves. The *sativa* species has in general up to thirteen long, slender, pronounced, jagged, spiky serrations, called fingers. Their color is typically a lighter shade of lime green. Leaves from the *indica* species are typically short and wide with seven to nine fat fingers. The color is usually a deep green.

The number of fingers also varies within the same species depending on environmental factors and where in the world the plant is grown. Lastly, the *ruderalis* species has typically three to five slender fingers on the thin leaves. Another reason for having different number of fingers has to do with the stage of development of the plant. Younger plants tend to have fewer fingers than mature plants.

Take Away Message

- Industrially grown hemp is currently used for a variety of products.
- No pesticides or herbicides are needed, making this an eco-friendly crop.
- Unfortunately, pesticides and herbicides are currently extensively used to grow hemp and marijuana.
- Hemp seeds are popular for their high nutrient content. They contain all nine essential amino acids.
- The omega-6 to omega-3 ratio in hemp seed oil is optimal for human health.
- Members of the genus *Cannabis*, including hemp and marijuana, typically are either male or female plants.
- Male plants and pollinated female plants are both low in cannabinoids.
- A properly pollinated female *Cannabis* plant will concentrate its entire energy to produce offspring, AKA hemp seeds.
- A non-pollinated female *Cannabis* plant will concentrate its entire energy on producing THC-containing resin.
- Fan leaves are the typical *Cannabis* leaves and are used globally in logos to represent marijuana.
- More cannabinoids and terpenes are produced in the flower compared to other parts such as the fan leaves.
- The *Cannabis* plant grows in two stages: the vegetative stage and the flowering stage.
- Once the plant enters the flowering stage, distinct male and female differences start to show.
- Cross-hybridization is the reason we have hundreds of different strains of this plant.
- The number of fingers on a leaf depends on a variety of factors.

Wanna Smoke Some Pot?

It is almost impossible to talk about hemp and CBD derived from hemp without mentioning marijuana and THC. Marijuana is the most commonly cultivated, trafficked, and abused illicit drug worldwide.[56] According to the World Health Organization (WHO), nearly 3% of the world population, meaning around 150 million individual users, consumes marijuana.

In 2014, approximately 22.2 million Americans 12 years of age or older reported current marijuana use, with 8.4% of this population reporting use within the previous month.[57] More men than women are consuming marijuana, and this gender gap widened in the years 2007 to 2014. Use is widespread in the adolescent and young adult population, and according to one survey, approximately 9% of eighth graders, and up to 35% of 12th graders, had consumed marijuana at least once.[58]

The United States Centers for Disease and Prevention (CDC) YRBS (Youth Risk Behavioral Surveillance) reported a lifetime use among U.S. high school students of 31.3% in 1991. This increased to 47.2% in 1999 and lowered slightly to 36.8% in 2009.[59] Other reports showed that approximately 43% of U.S. adults have tried marijuana, with 13% using it regularly.[60] In fact, the number of those who tried marijuana increased from 4% in 1969 to 43% in 2016.[61]

One way to estimate marijuana use, as well as use of other illicit drugs, in the general population is to analyze sewer water in different cities.[62] A study using this method in

19 European cities found that marijuana use was evenly distributed throughout Europe.[63]

For some, pot, weed, joint, marijuana, grass, cannabis, hemp, CBD, THC, herb, ganja, kaya, diesel, Mary Jane, bhang, cheeba, Dutchie, green, asparagus, cola, hash, hashish, dab, wax, shatter, crystals, or isolate are all the same. There are over 1,200 slang names describing the products from the *Cannabis* plant family.[64] Different cultures around the world have all their own names for this plant or plant product.

The name cannabis comes from the Greek word "kannabis" which was then translated into the Latin word cannabis. Prior to the use by Ancient Greeks, kannabis was originally used in the old Eastern European world as a Scythian or Thracian word.[65] In old Persia, it was known as Kanab. Centuries later it became the source for the English word canvas since long-lasting paper could be made from hemp. Cannabis may even have been mentioned in the Holy Bible as "kaneh-bosm", an ingredient in holy anointing oil.[66]

Other cultures described cannabis as Bhang (Hindi), Ganja (Sanskrit), Ma ren hua (China), Marihuana or Marijuana (Mexico and South American cultures), Mejorana chino (used in colloquial Spanish), Hashish (Arabia), Ma-kana (Bantu), or Weed (this expression first appeared as a synonym for "marijuana cigarette" around 1929, when more Americans started smoking "weed" as people looked for ways to feel uplifted at the twilight of The Roaring Twenties).[67] The word "weed" was then resurrected in the pop culture of the 80s together with the word "pot" or potiguaya which became popular in the 1930s in America.

Pot is a shortening of the Spanish potiguaya or potaguaya that came from potación de guaya, a wine or brandy in which marijuana buds have been steeped and is also known as "the drink of grief"[68].

Herbal marijuana has been used for thousands of years for medical purposes. Medical marijuana has its established place in the treatment of chronic cancer and neuropathic pain, multiple sclerosis, chemotherapy-induced nausea and vomiting, anorexia associated with weight loss in patients with acquired immune deficiency syndrome (AIDS), seizure control, elevated eye pressure such as in glaucoma, and headaches among others.[69,70,71,72,73,74]

I did not write this book to promote marijuana, whether as medical marijuana or as recreational substance. However, common sense dictates that we should look at such natural alternatives with overall fewer side effects compared to synthetic pharmacological solutions. In general, there is also a substantial cost saving to the patient and/or healthcare insurance companies when using marijuana compared to most pharmaceutical prescription drugs.

The two most common routes of marijuana consumption are inhalation and ingestion. When smoking, i.e. inhaling pot, the drug has a clear and fast path to the blood stream and effects can be experienced quickly. Bioavailability in the lung varies depending on the user. For example, chronic users are able to sustain the smoke in the lungs for a longer period of time compared to a naïve user.[75] Pulmonary assimilation of inhaled THC causes a maximum blood level within minutes. Psychotropic effects start within seconds to a few minutes, reach a maximum after 15-30 minutes, and taper off within two to three hours.[76]

Edible marijuana can take up to three hours or longer to take effect, depending on conditions such as an empty or full stomach. Other ways to consume marijuana are topical or sublingual applications.

Many people want us to believe that marijuana consumption is safe. However, according to medical literature, it has its dangers. It is well established that THC consumption impairs cognitive and motor function, and acute effects include paranoia and anxiety.[77] One group of scientists analyzed nine different studies about the effect of marijuana on driving skills and concluded that marijuana use by drivers is associated with a significantly increased risk of being involved in motor vehicle crashes.[78]

Another similar analysis studying 19 databases came to the exact same conclusion.[79] A study conducted in Canada found that 5% of drivers in fatal accidents were under the influence of marijuana.[80] A comparable study in France analyzing the data of over 10,000 fatal car crashes found that 8.8% of the drivers were under the influence of marijuana. A third of those drivers also had elevated alcohol levels in their blood.

A study looking at pilots' performances on flight stimulators found that marijuana enhanced visual and audial perception while impairing spatial orientation. However, all pilots showed a significant decrease in measurements of flying performance starting at about 30 minutes and lasting two hours after smoking marijuana. Deficits included increased risk of errors, altitude deviations, and poor alignment on landing.[81]

A similar study using nine pilots and a flight simulator was able to show that all nine pilots had a reduced performance up to 24 hours after smoking a moderate social dose of marijuana. However, only one of the pilots reported feeling the effects of the marijuana.[82]

Scientists were able to show, with imaging technology, that pot users had higher activity and blood flow in those parts of the brain associated with reward processing and decision-making. This led to a worse performance in financial decision-making while under the influence.[83] Very heavy marijuana users have persistent decision-making deficits and alterations in brain activity. Specifically, they may only focus on getting high while ignoring the negative consequences.[84]

A summary of adverse effects of recreational marijuana described the following problems associated with marijuana consumption: dependence, tolerance (getting used to a certain dose requiring a dose increase to obtain the same results), possible progression to other illicit drugs, impairment of cognition, impaired memory and psychomotor performance, a variety of psychiatric effects including precipitation and aggravation of schizophrenia, and physical health risks such as chronic bronchitis of the respiratory system.[85]

It is also noteworthy that several studies, as summarized by the National Institute on Drug Abuse,[86] described lasting brain damage or at least lasting changes in brain structures when using marijuana. Other scientists described that neuroimaging studies provided evidence of brain changes in areas that could affect cognition, logical processing, language processing, as well as balance of the body.[87]

Very mild side effects can sometimes be seen within six to 12 hours of consuming marijuana. The so-called hangover effect of marijuana includes cotton tongue, conjunctivitis, dizziness, psychosis, headaches, and fatigue. Dry mouth and dry tongue are cause by a decreased secretion by the salivary glands.

An animal study demonstrated that decreased secretion is a result of cannabinoid receptor activation in the various salivary glands of the oropharyngeal (mouth and throat) space.[88] In addition, direct effects of marijuana on receptors located in the brain cause a change in the activity of the autonomous nervous system (which controls involuntary functions), with decreased salivary secretion as result.[89] Cotton tongue is therefore the result of two distinct mechanisms, one being a local reaction while the other is a reaction in the central nervous system.

We know that predisposition for marijuana use and abuse involves both genetic as well as environmental factors.[90] The big question is whether marijuana consumption leads to the use of more aggressive and dangerous drugs.

One group of scientists conducted interviews with 226 marijuana users and found that the use of alcohol, tobacco, and/or marijuana might directly contribute to the initiation of new substance use.[91] Another study found that initiation of marijuana use typically follows alcohol use, but the reverse order also occurs and is more common for African-Americans than European-Americans. African-American women, for example, were nearly three times as likely as European-American women to initiate marijuana use before alcohol use.[92]

However, it could be shown that while alcohol use led to consumption of other drugs, patterns of marijuana use were not systematically related to intake of other substances.[93] And while one study clearly indicated that 44.7% of individuals with lifetime marijuana use progressed to other illicit drugs at some time in their lives, they also mentioned in the next sentence that sociodemographic characteristics, psychiatric disorders, and other indicators influence the decision to move up to stronger illegal drugs.[94]

In contrast to this study, The National Institute on Drug Abuse states that the majority of people who use marijuana do not go on to use other, "harder" substances.[95] This was confirmed by a study done by the Institute of Medicine, a branch of the National Academy of Sciences, in which it was revealed that there was no evidence that giving marijuana to sick people would increase illicit use in the general population. Nor is marijuana a "gateway drug" that prompts patients to use harder drugs like cocaine and heroin, the study said.[96]

This was confirmed by a study conducted with drug users in Amsterdam where the results indicated that personal characteristics, and not marijuana use, were the cause of changing from marijuana to cocaine.[97] This study included four surveys with almost 17,000 people and concluded that there was little difference in the probability of an individual taking up cocaine as to whether or not he or she had used marijuana.

All these facts support those who would like to legalize the use of CBD while keeping medical and recreational use of THC limited. Marijuana usage is associated with the potential for some degree of abuse and addiction. Nevertheless, public perception on this topic is rapidly changing.

Finally, I would like to add a few comments considering the ongoing opioid abuse epidemic. While both opioids and marijuana have the potential for abuse and dependency, there are significant differences between the two when it comes to mortality. The Center for Disease Control and Prevention (CDC) states that from 1999 to 2017, more than 700,000 people have died from a drug overdose.

In addition, around 68% of the 70,200+ drug overdose deaths in 2017 involved an opioid. And in 2017, the number of overdose deaths involving opioids (including prescription opioids and illegal opioids like heroin and illicitly manufactured fentanyl) was six times higher than in 1999.

On average, 130 Americans die every day from an opioid overdose.[98] Compared to these horrific mortality numbers from opioid abuse, marijuana use had little effect on non-AIDS mortality in men and on total mortality in women.[99] In fact, car accidents and lung cancer are the only domains where marijuana-attributable mortality is estimated to occur.[100]

The reason for the significant difference in mortality rates during opioid abuse versus marijuana abuse is the fact that the brain stem has very few receptors activated by THC compared to receptors that are activated by opium-like substances. The brain stem contains the centers for breathing, heart rate, blood pressure, and other important functions of the body. Opioids influence these very important centers, while marijuana will barely touch them.

In addition, the risk of developing a dependency on marijuana is much lower in comparison to opioids. In fact, opioid use is lower in states that eased marijuana laws.[101] One study showed that prescriptions filled for all opioids decreased by 2.11 million daily doses per year, from an average of 23.08 million daily doses per year, when a state instituted any medical marijuana law. Also, prescriptions for all opioids decreased by 3.742 million daily doses per year when medical marijuana dispensaries opened.[102]

As mentioned previously, this book is mainly about CBD. The brief information about THC-containing marijuana serves to highlight the significant differences between the two products. You will find plenty of research on the medical and/or recreational benefits, as well as the side effects, of marijuana, but providing more detailed information on THC-derived products goes beyond the scope of this book.

Take Away Message

- Marijuana is the most commonly cultivated, trafficked, and abused illicit drug worldwide.
- There are over 1,200 slang names describing the products from the *Cannabis* plant family.
- Herbal marijuana has been used for thousands of years for medical purposes.
- The two most common routes of marijuana consumption are inhalation and ingestion.
- THC consumption impairs cognitive and motor function, and acute effects include paranoia and anxiety.
- Pot users had higher activity and blood flow in those parts of the brain associated with reward processing and decision-making.
- Chronic marijuana use may change both the function as well as the structure of the human brain.
- Very mild side effects can sometimes be seen within six to 12 hours of consuming marijuana.
- Marijuana use was not systematically related to the consumption of other addictive substances.
- While both opioids and marijuana have the potential for abuse and dependency, there are significant differences between the two when it comes to mortality.

Hemp Versus Marijuana

Although CBD and psychoactive THC ultimately come from the same plant species, they are two distinct and different compounds with completely different effects on the human body.

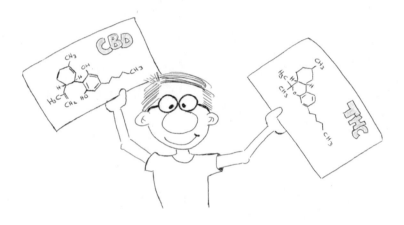

CBD versus THC

CBD

CBD, short for cannabidiol, is the second most prevalent of the active ingredients of *Cannabis*.[103] CBD has shown to have weak affinity (binding capacity) to CB1 and CB2 receptors.[104] CB receptors are so-called cannabinoid receptors found in our body.

Both CBD and THC are also known to bind to other receptors than just CB receptors.[105] Some of these receptors are called GPR55, GPR3, GPR6, GPR12, and GPR18, TRPV 1, TRPV 2, and TRPV 3, TRPA1 and

TRPM8, PPARγ, 5-HT1A, GABA, as well as α1-glycine and α3-glycine to name a few. Many of these will be explained later.

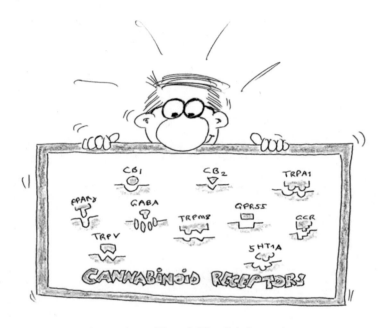

Some of our CB and CB-related receptors

CBD does not only influence brain function by directly binding to CB receptors, but rather works by influencing some of the enzymes used in the endocannabinoid system (ECS).

What is the ECS? It is an entire system in our body influenced by cannabinoid compounds such as CBD and THC. To make things more interesting, we also produce our own cannabinoid-like substances and enzymes regulating the cannabinoids from the plant and our own body. The endocannabinoid system is very complicated but will be clarified soon.

Why it is it named the endocannabinoid system? Early research first identified some cannabinoids in the plant *Cannabis*, then years later found a couple of receptors in the human body to which those cannabinoids attached. Thus, they were called cannabinoid receptors and the entire system was named the endocannabinoid system.

But as technology and science evolved over the past 50 years or so, many more receptors and other pieces of the system were found. Because researchers had already called it the endocannabinoid system, the name stuck, and we are now using it even though many more plant compounds, receptors, or even chemicals produced in our bodies are not directly related to the *Cannabis* plant.

CBD is a CB1 antagonist while THC is an CB1 agonist. This means that CBD can block a reaction when it attaches to CB1 receptors, while THC directly activates CB1 receptors, thereby creating a reaction inside the cell.

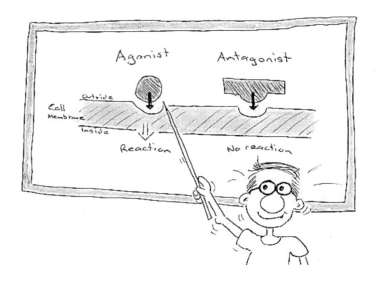

Agonists and antagonists

Why is that important? Because CBD has shown to diminish the psychotic effects of THC on the brain.[106,107,108,109] CBD decreased THC effects on brain regions involved in memory, anxiety and body temperature regulation.[110]

Researchers found that under certain conditions, such as being exposed for a prolonged amount of time to gastric acid, CBD can convert to THC.[111] While this was true in one animal study, the findings did not show to be relevant for humans as orally dosed CBD in doses yielding clinically relevant blood levels did not convert to THC.[112]

A comprehensive review of 132 original studies looked at the safety profile of CBD.[113] The authors found that physiological parameters such as heart rate, blood pressure, and body temperature are not altered by CBD.

Moreover, psychological and psychomotor functions are not adversely affected. The same holds true for gastrointestinal transit and food intake. Both CBD and THC have also proven to be good antioxidants.[114] In fact, CBD is a more potent antioxidant and free radical scavenger than Vitamin C or Vitamin E.[115]

To summarize, CBD works through different mechanisms such as attaching to CB receptors, by binding to or influencing other types of receptors, by inhibiting breakdown of enzymes, by exerting antioxidant properties, and via action by CBD metabolites. The use of CBD seems safe in both humans and animals.

THC

THC, short for delta-9-tetrahydrocannabinol, is the primary psychoactive constituent of marijuana.[116] Oral THC bioavailability, like with CBD, is only 6-10% due to gastric degradation and extensive first-pass metabolism in the liver.

First-pass effect describes the mechanism by which compounds absorbed from the gut go first through the liver before being distributed to other places in the body. When passing through the liver, they can be changed or degraded to the point that they lose most of their effectiveness. Sometimes, the changed compound is more active than the original absorbed ingredient.

THC rapidly oxidizes to its active metabolite 11-hydroxy-THC (11-OH-THC).[117] When smoked, THC is quickly absorbed through the lungs and swiftly reaches high concentration in the blood.[118] Inhalation through the lungs prevents the first-pass metabolism in the liver.

The adverse effects of THC include impaired short-term memory making it difficult to learn and to retain information, impaired motor coordination interfering with driving skills and increasing the risk of injuries, and altered judgment increasing the risk of sexual behaviors that facilitate the transmission of sexually transmitted diseases. When THC is used chronically, addiction occurs in about 9% of users overall, 17% of those who begin use in adolescence, and 25 to 50% of those who are daily users.

Other adverse effects of THC include altered brain development, poor educational outcome with increased likelihood of dropping out of school, cognitive impairment with lower IQ among those who were frequent users during adolescence, and diminished life satisfaction and achievement.

Medical consequences include symptoms of chronic bronchitis and an increased risk of chronic psychosis disorders (including schizophrenia) in persons with a predisposition to such disorders, and in high doses, paranoia and psychosis.[119]

On the other hand, THC has also shown to have positive effects as well. One study revealed that 97% of marijuana users took it primarily for chronic pain. They reported a 64% decrease in pain. Half of all respondents also noted relief from stress/anxiety, and 45% reported relief from insomnia.[120] Other authors reported benefits in nausea and vomiting as well as appetite stimulation in anorexia.[121]

Other studies demonstrated the usefulness of THC in cancer patients with a whopping 96% of the patients reporting improvement of their symptoms.[122] The authors concluded that THC from marijuana is a palliative treatment for cancer patients that is well tolerated, effective, and safe to help patients cope with the malignancy related symptoms.

One review analyzed trials involving medical marijuana for neurological disorders and reported that although trials with positive findings were identified for anorexia nervosa, anxiety, PTSD, psychotic symptoms, agitation in Alzheimer's disease and dementia, Huntington's disease, Tourette syndrome, and dyskinesia in Parkinson's disease, definitive conclusions on its efficacy could not yet be drawn.[123]

Medical and scientific literature is vast when it comes to THC. Many books have been written about marijuana and its main psychoactive compound delta-9-tetrahydrocannabinol. However, this book is about CBD and mainly how it can be used together with other plant extracts such as essential oils. Please refer to other sources if you want to learn more about the effects of THC.

Do You Need to Add A Little THC For CBD To Work?

Whether one needs to add a little THC to CBD to experience the full benefit depends likely on what one wants to achieve or experience. Many of the immediate effects of CBD cannot be felt since CBD is not a hallucinogenic and does create the feeling of a "high." One cannot feel an immediate balancing effect on the immune system, for example.

There is no question that the consumption of full-spectrum CBD or the consumption of a CBD/THC blend will benefit from the entourage effect, which will be explained in further detail later. That could be an explanation why many believe that they need to add some THC to the CBD for it to work, but there is currently insufficient evidence to support that notion.

On the other hand, there seems to be good evidence that adding CBD to THC may be beneficial. Most clinical studies have shown that CBD in fact inhibits the psychoactive effects of THC. CBD also blocks the formation of 11-hydroxy-tetrahydro-cannabinol (11-OH-THC), the most psychoactive metabolite of THC.[124]

CBD was found to potentiate some therapeutic effects of THC such as cancer growth inhibition,[125] while counteracting most of its undesirable effects such as sedation, psychotropic effects, tachycardia, abnormally increased appetite for food, thus allowing the use of higher and more efficacious co-administered doses of THC. While CBD is demonstrated to antagonize some undesirable effects of THC, it does contribute to its analgesic, anti-emetic, and anti-carcinogenic properties.[126]

Take Away Message

- CBD and THC are two distinct and different compounds with completely different effects on the human body.
- There is an entire system in our body influenced by the two most commonly found cannabinoid compounds (CBD and THC) in the *Cannabis* plant, called the endocannabinoid system (ECS).
- CBD works through different mechanisms such as attaching to CB receptors, attaching or influencing other types of receptors, by inhibiting breakdown enzymes, by exerting antioxidant properties, and via action by CBD metabolites.
- The use of CBD seems safe in both humans and animals.
- There is insufficient evidence to support the notion that a little THC is needed to improve the way CBD works.
- CBD was found to potentiate some therapeutic effects of THC such as cancer growth inhibition, while counteracting most of its undesirable effects.
- The fact that CBD lowers some of potentially undesired effects of THC permitted the administration of higher doses of THC when combined with CBD.

Seed to Seal

Hemp is a fiber-generating plant with well-known antibacterial performance.[127] Hemp fibers are especially attractive due to their natural antibacterial property.[128]

Hemp and marijuana plants contain powerful antibacterial agents. For example, all five major cannabinoids including cannabidiol, cannabichromene, cannabigerol, Δ9-THC, and cannabinol showed potent activity against methicillin-resistant staphylococcus aureus (MRSA) bacteria.[129]

The inhibitory effect of hemp on bacterial growth expands also to fungi such as *Candida*.[130] However, investigators found elevated fungal spore concentrations in indoor grown cultures.[131] The antimicrobial nature of the hemp/ marijuana plant theoretically obviates the need for major pesticides and herbicides. But since growing marijuana is illegal in the US and its market value is so great, many growers started to secretly use some chemicals, typically synthetic fertilizers and pesticides, to feed and protect the crop from microbial and animal infestation and improve their yields.[132]

It is mentioned in medical literature that the lack of Environmental Protection Agency (EPA) regulations and absence of approved chemical products for supporting the growth of marijuana may result in consumer exposures to hazardous pesticides or higher residue levels.[133] Some authors declared that a public safety threat has arisen relating to application of pesticides on marijuana plants with intensified toxicity in concentrated products of particular concern.[134]

In fact, the following toxic chemicals have been found in both medical and recreational marijuana products: pesticides such as bifenthrin, chlorpyrifos, diazinon, methamidophos, and teflubenzuron; fungicides such as tebuconazole; growth regulators such as ethephon, as well as mosquito repellants such as DEET and malathion.[135]

There are potential problems with heavy metal contamination of hemp and marijuana products. Reports have shown that marijuana has been intentionally contaminated with metals like lead to increase the market weight. This may have dire consequences. In 2008 for example, 150 people in Germany suffered from lead poisoning as the result of using manually adulterated marijuana.[136]

But heavy metals are also found in the soil of hemp and marijuana fields. The plants are known to effectively absorb heavy metals such as cadmium and copper from contaminated soils. In fact, one author called hemp and marijuana plants "bio-accumulators" because they recruit heavy metals such as lead, mercury, cadmium, and arsenic from the soil into the plant biomass. While this can be used to decontaminate bad soil, it is at the same time a liability if hemp and marijuana grown in such media is used in the production of CBD and THC consumables.[137]

Also, solvents used in the preparation and extraction of CBD might be left over in the products. In fact, one study looked at pesticide and solvent residues in products containing CBD and/or THC and found a considerable amount of residual solvent and pesticide contamination in over 80% of the samples.[138] Even more worrisome is the fact that up to 69.5% of pesticide and chemical residues make it into the smoke of marijuana products and are being inhaled by consumers. The authors of that study correctly concluded that the exposures to marijuana users are substantial and that this may pose a significant toxicological threat.[139]

Another study showed that 85% of the samples used in their analysis tested positive for pesticides. Many harbored multiple contaminants including 24 distinct pesticide agents of every class. Among them were insecticides, miticides, fungicides, insecticidal synergists and growth regulators, organophosphates, organochlorides, carbamates, carbaryl, boscalid, bifenazate, pyraclostrobin, fenpyroximate, and myclobutanil, with documented associated toxicities like carcinogens, neurotoxins, cholinesterase inhibitors, developmental and reproductive toxins, and endocrine disruptors.[140]

It is also necessary to understand the basics of cannabinoid extraction and preparation, as different techniques are used in this industry. Hemp material can either be pressed, CO_2 extracted, lipid extracted, or solvent extracted.

A good method to extract pure CBD from plant material is a technique using pressurized supercritical CO_2 which removes volatile oils from hemp while leaving no solvent residue(s). When pressure is applied and the temperature is lowered, CO_2 can become a liquid. Once the liquid is created, the temperature is raised again to create the supercritical phase.[141] Presently, high-quality CBD is most likely obtained through this type of carbon dioxide (CO_2) extraction.[142]

This supercritical CO_2 is then mixed with the plant material, and by doing so it pulls the compounds out of the plant. Then, the solution passes through a separator chamber in which the desired parts can be salvaged, while the CO_2 continues into a condensation chamber. The main advantage of this method over using solvents is that it is non-toxic and non-flammable. The CO_2 can be recycled or released into the atmosphere.

After the CO_2 extraction, the solution is subjected to winterization. In this process, organic solvent, usually ethyl alcohol (EtOH), is used to remove the cannabinoids from the black gooey mass obtained from the CO_2 extraction. The organic solvent fraction is purified (to get the CBD) using distillation or flash chromatography.

Some home growers of marijuana plants select to use cheap and simple methods to extract plant materials, like mixing either olive oil, coconut oil, or even melted butter with the plant material. Before the material is combined with the oil, it must be decarboxylated since the carboxylated form is not very potent.

In other words, the acid precursors of THC and CBD, naturally present in the plants, need to have CO_2 removed for the THC or CBD to be activated properly. This can be done by exposing the plant material to light and heat. It is typically heated to 250 to 300° Fahrenheit for 30 to 60 minutes. Once this process is complete, the carrier oil is added and heated again for a couple of hours. It is a simple method, but it has a low yield of high-quality CBD.

Another method is to use solvents. They are often used during the extraction process in order to create highly concentrated products. Once the solvents do their job, they evaporate. However, evaporation might be incomplete and result in contamination of the end product.

Solvents might include ethanol, benzene, hexane, naphtha, petroleum ether, low-grade alcohols, butane, and olive oil. They all can pose a significant risk of toxic chemical concentration. Hexane and benzene for example are neurotoxic, and naptha and petroleum ether are both potential carcinogens. In some countries, naphtha is equivalent to diesel or kerosene fuel.

Ethanol also extracts chlorophyll which may lead to an unpleasant taste unless the material obtained is carefully filtered to remove undesired plant material. Pure ethanol extraction is cheaper than supercritical CO_2 extraction and is still used by many companies today.[143] Cold pressing as an extraction method is only used to obtain oil from hemp seeds. This method will not allow for any meaningful CBD extraction.

Hemp and marijuana plant material is usually preheated or stored for a prolonged amount of time in order to decarboxylate the acidic cannabinoids, as mentioned earlier. The downside of the heating process is that the higher the temperature used, the more of the volatile terpenes (mostly monoterpenes such as terpineol, myrcene, β-pinene, and terpinolene) are lost.[144] The use of olive oil as solvent seems to have the advantage of better preserving these kinds of terpenes.[145] The downside of prolonged storage is that the plant material is at risk of contamination with bacteria, fungi, or other types of microorganisms.

I personally like to use pure CBD isolate powder obtained by supercritical CO_2 extraction. Not only does CO_2 completely evaporate once the pressure is released, it is also non-toxic. As I mentioned in other chapters of this book, the downside of this CO_2 extracted powder is that it does not contain any terpenes and therefore loses what we call the entourage effect (described in detail later). This however can be mitigated by mixing the CBD powder with essential oils, which is one of the reasons why I am writing this book.

The CBD and Essential Oil combination opens an entirely new world with countless possibilities to benefit from all these compounds simultaneously. If you have never been introduced to either CBD or essential oils and would like to begin using this wonderful combo, my team and I will be happy to guide you in your wellness, beauty, and health journey. At the end of this book is more information on how to contact us.

In some cases, hemp and marijuana processing includes gamma-irradiation for sterilization. While no remaining radiation could be found in the end products, studies have shown that radiation changes the terpene content of the products while leaving CBD, THC, as well as water content of the products unchanged.[146] One study showed that gamma irradiation did produce a 10% decrease in β-caryophyllene, a very important sesquiterpene found in CBD.[147]

The good news in all of this is that CBD can be derived from plants industrially grown outdoors and hence has a slightly diminished risk of being contaminated by highly toxic chemicals used indoors. Most of the studies demonstrating herbicide, pesticide, fungicide, and fertilizer contamination are from marijuana cultures and not industrial hemp fields.

But that does not mean that you can let your guard down. As mentioned earlier, many hemp growers use fertilizer, pesticides, and herbicides, all of which can end up in the CBD products. Even if grown completely without toxic chemicals, some of these dangerous substances are used later in the processing of the plant and can still make it into your CBD products. It is buyer beware.

Know the source, know the company, and also know the type of CBD product being bought, since certain extraction methods do not use chemicals at all and others leave toxic solvents in the product.

Make sure that the hemp plants are organic and sustainably grown. They should not have been treated with heavy metals or commercial toxins while growing on the fields or during the processes of extraction and preparation of the final product. Make sure the product is tested thoroughly.

If you choose to smoke pot, you want to make sure that you are consuming clean marijuana, since over 80% of the commercially available marijuana products are contaminated and may cause acute lung toxicity or chronic lung damage including lung cancer.[148]

Seed to Seal certification is extremely important for essential oils, and the same quality assurance process is also of the outmost importance for CBD. Make sure that your CBD seller has all of this in place and under control. Be aware that anyone can write "organic" or "certified," so source your CBD from someone you know and trust.

Take Away Message
- Hemp and marijuana plants are known to contain powerful antibacterial agents.
- Since growing marijuana is mostly illegal in the U.S. and its market value is so great, many growers started to secretly use synthetic fertilizers and pesticides to feed and protect their crops.
- Toxic chemicals have been found in both medical and recreational marijuana.
- There is also a problem with heavy metal contamination of hemp and marijuana products.
- Solvents in the preparation and extraction of CBD might be left over in the products.
- Hemp material can either be pressed, CO_2 extracted, lipid extracted, or solvent extracted.
- Pressurized supercritical CO_2 extracts volatile oils from *Cannabis* while leaving no residues.
- Some home growers of marijuana plants use cheap and simple methods to extract plant materials.
- Solvents are often used during the extraction process in order to create highly concentrated products.
- Cold pressing as an extraction method is only used to obtain oil from hemp seeds.
- Hemp and marijuana plant material is usually preheated or stored for a prolonged amount of time in order to decarboxylate the acidic cannabinoids.

- The CBD-Essential Oil combination opens an entirely new world with countless possibilities to benefit from all these compounds simultaneously.
- CBD can be derived from plants industrially grown outdoors without fertilizers, pesticides, or herbicides.
- Know the source, know the company, and know the type of CBD product being bought, since certain extraction methods do not use chemicals at all.
- Seed to Seal certification is extremely important for essential oils, and the same quality assurance process is also of the outmost importance for CBD.

Part 2: Science and the Body

The Endocannabinoid System

The endocannabinoid system is composed of receptors (keyholes), ligands (keys), and enzymes controlling the synthesis and degradation of endocannabinoids (construction cranes and hammers), as well as endocannabinoid transporters (boats).[149]

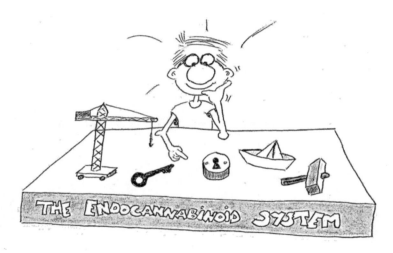

The endocannabinoid system

Specific information about each of these parts and how they all work together will be explained in detail soon, but the ECS as a whole should be addressed first. The main purpose of the ECS is to protect multiple organ systems and to keep them in good balance, called homeostasis. The importance of the ECS is much more significant for a healthy body than previously thought.

The ECS has homeostatic roles in hunger, appetite and energy metabolism, neural plasticity (formation of brain pathways) and neuroprotection, pain modulation, memory, the flight or fight response, connective tissue repair, thermoregulation, stress, anxiety, sleep, immune response, as well as human behavior. Basically, the ECS involves homeostasis with regards to relaxation, eating, sleeping, forgetting, and protecting.[150]

A dysfunctional or suboptimal functioning ECS has been connected to a variety of conditions such as irritable bowel syndrome,[151] fibromyalgia,[152] migraines,[153] schizophrenia,[154] uncontrolled Parkinson's,[155] Huntington's disease,[156] chronic motion sickness,[157] anorexia and bulimia,[158] and possibly obesity.[159] In fact, the terms "ECS deficiency syndrome" or "clinical endocannabinoid deficiency syndromes CEDS" have been now created to describe some of these pathological conditions.[160]

So, beneficial effects of the ECS have been described in pathological conditions such as nausea and vomiting, inflammation, pain, post-traumatic stress disorder (PTSD), autoimmune diseases such as multiple sclerosis (MS), thyroid disorders, and rheumatoid arthritis, cardiovascular disorders such as strokes, autism, cancer, neurological diseases such as dementia and Alzheimer's, Parkinson's, Huntington's, schizophrenia, psychosis, depression, panic attacks, anxiety, and obsessive compulsive behavior, insomnia, obesity, anorexia, metabolic disorders, epilepsy, and glaucoma.[161]

Knowing that this ECS is responsive to many plants, their extracts, and their essential oils should give us pause and let us admire the treasures of nature that were at least partly created to support humans and animals alike.

It is also interesting to mention that neither CBD nor THC were the first cannabinoid discovered by scientists. In 1855, the Pharmaceutical Society of Paris awarded a prize to a scientist for the "good analysis of hemp" but unfortunately the compound discovered at that time was an impure volatile sesquiterpene and not one of the important cannabinoids. [162]

Many other scientists of the time tried to isolate and define structures of compounds obtained from the *Cannabis* plant. Cannabinol (CBN) was the first cannabinoid discovered and isolated at the end of the 19th century. Its chemical structure was established in the early 1930s and its chemical synthesis first achieved in 1940. It was during that same year that CBD was first described in scientific literature.[163]

Two years later, in 1942, a group of researchers discovered and isolated THC for the first time.[164] It still took another 20-some years and the emergence of newer technologies to finally fully analyze the complete chemical structure and stereochemistry of CBD, which was then reported in an article in 1963.[165]

Research on phytocannabinoids (cannabinoids from plants) intensified after these discoveries, but it was not until 1990 that endocannabinoid receptors were properly described.[166] The current state of research and understanding supports the idea that CB1 receptors mostly modulate neurological functions, while CB2 receptors are more responsible for immune modulation.

The last few years have shown a remarkable increase in research activity and publications on CBD, mainly stimulated by the discovery of its anti-inflammatory, antioxidative, and neuroprotective effects.[167] These studies have suggested a wide range of possible therapeutic effects of CBD on conditions such as strokes, neurodegenerative diseases (Parkinson's disease, Alzheimer's disease), diabetes, rheumatoid arthritis, other inflammatory diseases, as well as nausea and cancer.

Let's discuss each component of the endocannabinoid system (ECS) and how they work. It is a daunting task as the ECS is much more complicated than originally assumed and new research emerges almost on a monthly basis. At first the information may seem very science-y and complicated, but there will be a summary of the current knowledge in simple terms at the end of this chapter.

Soon you will understand that the ECS can be influenced and improved by augmenting endocannabinoid biosynthesis, by decreasing endocannabinoid and phytocannabinoid degradation, and by augmenting or decreasing receptor density or function via a healthy lifestyle.

Cannabinoid Receptors

Cannabinoid receptors can be found all over the human body. Of the many receptors involved in the ECS, the most abundant are G-protein receptors known as CB1 and CB2, and there may even be a CB3, CB4, and CB5 as well. And while these receptors are mostly expressed in different tissues, they can also coexist at the same location.[168]

G-protein-coupled receptors are a class of receptors that have an "inbox" on the surface of a cell. This inbox or mailbox can receive emails or letters that then initiate a reaction on the inside of the cell membrane.

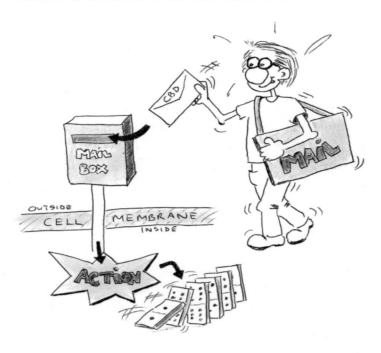

The workings of G-protein-coupled receptors

These G-protein-coupled receptors are made of a single polypeptide (short protein) that is folded into a specific shape and embedded in a cell's membrane. They are called G-protein-coupled receptors because they are very close to a class of proteins on the inside of the cell membrane, we call G-proteins.

Once they activate these G-proteins, something will change on the inside of the cell membrane and one or more signals are passed on to the other proteins within the cell. Activation of a single G-protein can affect the production of hundreds or even thousands of what we call second messenger molecules, like the dominoes in the picture.[169]

Second messenger molecules are what the name describes. They take the primary information and pass it on as a second messenger to other parts of the cell. Putting a "letter into the mailbox" on the outside of the cell membrane, starts a reaction that ends up having a domino effect inside the cell.

Receptors can be very specific, meaning that only a certain substance, or ligand, can attach to the receptor. Other receptors can bind several types of ligands that look very similar and are therefore less specific receptors.

Overall, activation of CB1 receptors often results in reduction of neuropathic pain as well as diminished nausea and vomiting. Suppression of CB1 receptors leads to a decrease in food intake but an increase in depressive disorders. On the other hand, activation of CB2 receptors leads to decreased amount of bone loss, deceased inflammation, as well as a decrease in neuropathic pain while at the same time supporting the immune system.

CBD and the activation of mostly CB2 receptors can either enhance or suppress immune function. This strange duality of action just highlights the main reason for having an ECS in the first place: to create homeostasis in various body systems and organs including the immune system.

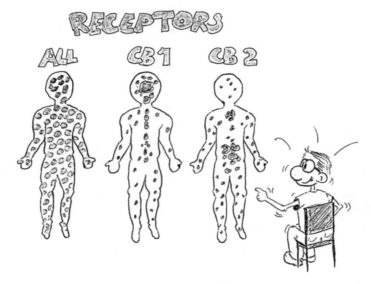

CB1, CB2, and other cannabinoid-like receptors

CB1 Receptors

CB1 receptors are mostly found in the central nervous system, but also to a lesser extent in the uterus, testes, gut, adrenal glands, heart, lungs, prostate, adipose tissue, ovaries, bone marrow, thymus, tonsils, and elsewhere. They impact several neurotransmitters, including GABA, glutamate, dopamine, and serotonin.

Neurotransmitters are chemicals produced in the body with the purpose to transmit certain signals once they attach to their receptors in the brain and the nerves. Activation of CB1 receptors promotes the psychoactive effects of cannabinoids.

CB1 is the most abundant G-protein-coupled receptor expressed in the brain, with particularly dense occurrence in areas important for reward processing, movement, memory, emotions, survival instincts, sex drive, as well as thinking, perceiving, producing, and understanding language.[170]

Researchers found that cannabinoid receptor binding sites in the human brain are localized mainly in the forebrain areas associated with higher cognitive functions, forebrain, midbrain as well as hindbrain areas associated with the control of movement, and in hindbrain areas associated with the control of motor and sensory functions of the autonomic nervous system. But as mentioned earlier, CB1 receptors are also found outside the brain and nervous system tissue.

CB2 Receptors

CB2 receptors are particularly abundant in peripheral tissues of the immune system (leukocytes, spleen, lymph nodes, tonsils, thymus, bone marrow) and the gastrointestinal system. To a lesser extent they are also found in the central nervous system. In fact, CB2 expression levels in the immune tissue are 10 to 100-fold higher than that of CB1.[171] We now know that human leukocytes are rich in CB2 receptor expression.[172] Leukocytes are blood cells that play an important role in the body's immune system.

How are certain commands, embedded in your genetic code, carried out? Let me start with an example: Once upon a time there was a village. In that village there was a bank. In that bank there was a vault, and, in that vault, there was a book with secret codes. Doctor Oli opened the book and looked at a page with secret symbols representing commands for the cell to produce certain things. But because that one page could not be removed from the bank, it had to be copied using a copy machine. For every command that was copied from the page, the copy machine produced a little note.

Doctor Oli then grabbed the phone and called a trucking company. He relayed the individual commands copied onto the little paper notes to the various drivers of the trucks. The trucks were all loaded with different materials. It was very important to get the sequence of the commands in correct order. The trucks then drove the different truck loads in correct sequence to a manufacturing plant.

Once they arrived, the trucks unloaded, and the manufacturing plant workers assembled the materials in the order they arrived. And this is how the commands originally hidden in a book stored away in a bank were executed. In your body, this is how a cell creates hormones or receptors for example.

The village is a cell. The bank is the nucleus of the cell where the genetic information is stored. The book with secret codes is our genetic information contained in a double-chained helix called deoxyribonucleic acid (DNA). The copy made from the one page is called ribonucleic acid (RNA). The little copied notes are called messenger RNA or simply mRNA. They each carry a command that is being transmitted to the trucking company. The trucks are called transfer RNA or tRNA, and the truck loads are individual amino acids. The trucks now drive to the manufacturing plant we call ribosomes.

Depending on the order of arrival at the manufacturing plant, the tRNA will unload their individual amino acids which will then be added to the assembly line. As more trucks arrive and unload their amino acids, the chain of amino acids gets longer and longer until no more trucks arrive. The chain of amino acids is now large enough to be called a polypeptide or even a protein.

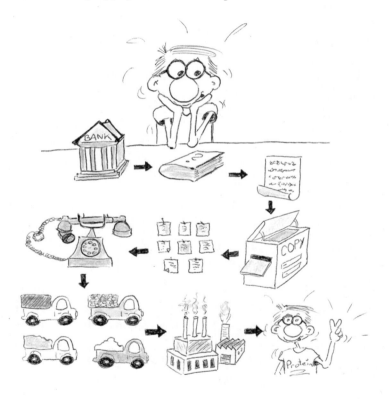

How genetic commands are carried out

This entire process was initiated by the code contained in the DNA and copied to the RNA, a process we call transcription. The process of assembling the amino acids in a specific order is then called translation of the genetic information. And this is how a cell knows what to do.

Now let's go back to CB2 receptors and immune cells. How does the cell know whether to create CB1 or CB2 receptors or other things? The basic information and commands for the creation/expression of these receptors is contained in the DNA. Depending on several factors such as overall health, lifestyle, and need for support in specific systems such as the immune system, the cell will know what part of the DNA to copy into RNA and then create smaller pieces of mRNA which then use tRNA to assemble proteins that for example make CB2 receptors on the surface of immune cells if they need it.

The fact that many immune cells contain CB2 receptors highlights the important role of phytocannabinoids such as CBD as well as endocannabinoids (those cannabinoids created by your own body) in the proper functioning of the immune system.

In general, receptors do not stay forever at their location on the cell membranes. They can be upregulated and downregulated, meaning they can be constantly added or removed depending on the need of the cells or organ systems. So, the creation (expression) and removal (degradation) of receptors is in constant flux. In fact, recent studies have demonstrated that CB2 is expressed within the central nervous system mostly in times of inflammation of the brain tissue.[173]

CB3 Receptors

CB3 receptors have not yet been officially classified as such. However, there is ample evidence that GPR55, a G-protein-coupled receptor, is a cannabinoid receptor distinct from CB1 and CB2.[174,175,176,177,178,179] This receptor type can be found in the brain (especially in the cerebellum which is the "small brain" in charge of balance and motor function), the spinal cord, and the gut.[180]

GPR55 receptors have also been found in the bones. Research demonstrated the ability of these bone receptors to suppress osteoclast formation but stimulate osteoblast function.[181] Osteoclasts are responsible for bone removal while osteoblasts stimulate bone growth. Therefore, receptor activation stimulates bone formation and suppresses bone resorption.[182]

Cannabinoids are also produced within synovial tissues around the joints, and preclinical studies have shown that cannabinoid receptor ligands, like CBD, are effective in the treatment of inflammatory arthritis.[183] It is also noteworthy that endocannabinoids are produced in the bone marrow and therefore play a direct role in the regulation of bone formation and degradation.[184] Overall, CBD's ability to activate cannabinoid bone and joint receptors, such as the potential CB3 receptor GPR55, plays an important role in bone mass and the regulation of bone disease.[185]

Other CB-like Receptors

Other ECS-related receptors include GPR19, GPR 119, PPAR receptors, TRPV receptors, α3-Glycine receptors, serotonin receptors such as 5-HTA, and GABA-A receptors. This list is likely not complete, and research in the very near future will describe more of these receptors and the function they fulfill in our bodies. This is all much more complicated than just talking about a couple of receptors like CB1 and CB2 activated by either CBD or THC or other similar compounds.

How do CB Receptors Work?

As you read earlier, G-protein receptors are part of a large protein family of receptors that detect molecules outside of the cell membranes, and when properly activated by the binding of these molecules they will undergo a change in structure.[186] This change in structure leads to the activation of subunits on the inside of the cell membrane which then in turn will trigger a cascade of events within the cell called a cellular response.

Our cell membranes also contain channels that can be opened or closed depending on the signals they receive. When some of these channels open, electrolytes such as calcium can enter the cell. This can change the electric balance across the cell membrane which in turn initiates an effect on the inside of the cell.[187] Such an effect could be the release of neurotransmitters, for example. The nerves in our brain work by combining electrical signals that travel on the outside of the nerve sheath with chemical signals that are generated at the synaptic cleft. But what is a synaptic cleft?

Our nerves don't really touch each other. There is a tiny gap between the part where one nerve ends and where the other starts. This small space is the synaptic cleft or gap, and the entire tiny area is a synapse.

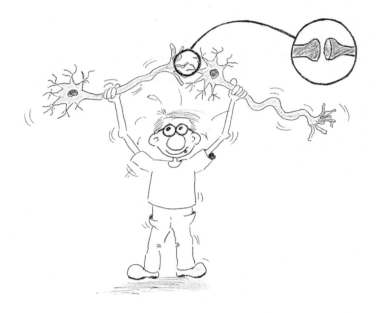

How nerves connect to each other

The end of the first nerve is called a terminal button and is the pre-synaptic part of the gap. The beginning of the next nerve is called a dendrite and is the post-synaptic part of the gap.

So once an electric signal reaches the terminal button it cannot just jump over to the next dendrite. It needs something to cross the tiny synaptic cleft. So, our body generates neurotransmitters to fulfill this function.

Electric signals coming down a nerve (or alternatively, a ligand such as CBD or THC binding to receptors where the nerve cell ends) causes a reaction that releases or inhibits the release of neurotransmitters (typically stored in little bubbles on the terminal button) into the synaptic cleft.

The released neurotransmitters then cross the synaptic cleft. Once a neurotransmitter finds the appropriate receptor on the other side of this narrow space, a new electrical signal is generated, and the brain and nerve signals can continue to spread.

Some neurotransmitters are created in the gut wall. This is one of the reasons why a healthy gut is crucial for good brain function.

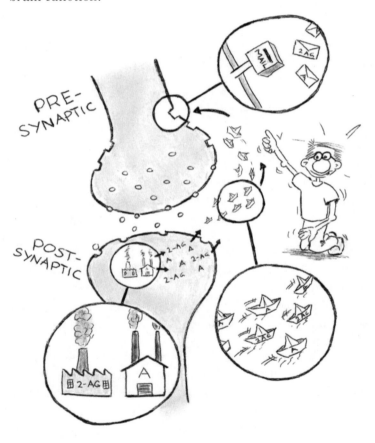

A synapse with all its parts including CB receptors

Another way to influence the release or inhibition of the release of neurotransmitters at the synapse comes from our own endocannabinoid system. The postsynaptic part of the synapse contains little manufacturing plants including all the enzymes necessary to produce our endocannabinoids anandamide and 2-arachidonoyl-glycerol (2-AG). You will read more about these two very soon. They are released on demand if the need for homeostasis arises. Homeostasis is a state of balance indicating health and wellness of the various organ systems and of a person as a whole.

Once released, they need to cross the synaptic gap backwards to reach the endocannabinoid receptors on the presynaptic nerve ending. Because they are fatty by nature, they will need transporters to get them across the watery gap. These transporters are like little boats, and they unload the endocannabinoids in form of letters at the presynaptic harbors.

The letters find their way into the appropriate mailboxes (CB1, CB2, and other cannabinoid receptors) and once the letters are received, something will change on the inside of the presynaptic part. This is how our own endocannabinoids but also phytocannabinoids interact with the information passed on from one nerve to the next.

Activation of CB1 and CB2 receptors in the brain for example may cause opposite reactions. That helps to explain why THC is hallucinogenic, or in other words gives you a high, and CBD on the other hand reduces the feeling of being high. Depending on the organ system, there are either similar or completely opposite effects when CB1 and CB2 receptors are activated.

In the gut, activation of CB1 and CB2 receptors results in the same effects like decreased bowel motility, reduced inflammation in the gut wall, and enhanced permeability for food.

On the other hand, in the liver, activation of CB1 and CB2 receptors have opposite effects. CB1 activation results in increased steatosis (accumulation of fat in the liver) and fibrogenesis (formation of fibers in the liver ultimately leading to a scarred or cirrhotic liver), hepatic apoptosis (induction of cell death in the liver), as well as hepatic proliferation (increased creation of new liver cells in order to try to limit liver damage) in the liver tissue. CB2 activation has exactly the opposite effect and as a result, promotes better liver function.[188]

Most books or lectures describe the effects of cannabinoids on the brain, often only discussing the mechanisms of CB1 receptors. But it is very important to also understand CB2 receptors and their effects on the body. I already mentioned that CB2 receptors are mainly found on immune cells. The immune system is a very complicated and delicate system. It creates two different type of responses against attacks on the human body: the innate and the acquired, or adaptive, immune responses.

The innate system is like a first line of defense while the adaptive system is way more sophisticated. Certain immune cells in your body do not need prior exposure to know that a specific substance is an enemy and that defenses have to be created to guard against that opponent. These types of immune cells are always ready to fight whatever comes their way. These are the cells of the innate immune system.

On the other hand, the human adaptive immune system includes cells that are involved in a response against specific threats. It involves white blood cells known as B-lymphocytes and T-lymphocytes. These kinds of cells are like the SWAT team of defense cells.

B-type cells are bone marrow or bursa-derived whereas T-type cells also come from the bone marrow but then migrate to the thymus, a small organ behind your sternum or breastbone, where they then mature. Adaptive immune cells remember foreign invaders after their first encounter and fight them off the next time they enter the body.

B-cells fight bacteria and viruses by making Y-shaped proteins called antibodies, which are specific to each pathogen and lock onto the surface of an invading cell and mark it for destruction by other immune cells. [189]

So, B-cells attack invaders outside the cells before they can infect, while T-cells kill invaders inside the cells after infection. Humoral (blood) immunity depends on the B-cells, while cellular immunity depends on the T-cells. [190]

When CBD attaches to CB2 receptors on immune cells, an immunosuppressive effect occurs which includes suppressed cytokine (inflammatory chemicals) production. CBD-mediated immune suppression includes humoral immunity (B-cells) and cellular immunity (T-cells). [191,192] Why is the suppression of the immune system sometimes a good thing?

Often, the immune system goes into overdrive and as a result, we suffer from significant inflammation or even autoimmune diseases where the body's own tissues are attacked in what could be referred to as friendly fire. Regulating these processes and controlling inflammation is therefore a good thing. There is now a large body of evidence indicating that the activation of CB2 receptors is linked to a variety of immune events including protection of neuroinflammation.[193] CB2 has also been shown to modulate the function of all immune cell types.[194]

To summarize, CB1 and CB2 cannabinoid receptors are mostly located in different parts of our body and work through different mechanisms. Recent evidence suggests that there are more CB receptors called CB3, CB4, and CB5 receptors. The discovery in the early 1990s of these specific membrane receptors for marijuana led to the identification of an entire endogenous signaling system in our body, now known as the endocannabinoid system (ECS).

Binding to CB receptors cause either an increase or a decrease of neurotransmitters released into the synaptic gap. Depending on this mechanism, signal transmission between nerves can either be facilitated or slowed down.

As a result, certain reactions in the body can be activated or inhibited. We believe today that this entire endocannabinoid system serves the function of homeostasis, meaning to balance reactions within the body. The ECS allows us to balance multiple systems in our body and hence to improve wellness and overall health.

Cannabinoid Ligands

If the receptor is a keyhole, a ligand is the key. Putting the correct key into a keyhole either opens the door (agonist) or prevents it from being opened because there is now a key in the keyhole (antagonist). It is the same with ligands and receptors. If you get the correct ligand to bind to the appropriate receptor a reaction will occur, either activation or inhibition.

There are three kinds of cannabinoid ligands: Endocannabinoids which are produced within the human body, phytocannabinoids which are produced in plants, and synthetic cannabinoids which are produced in a lab.

Endocannabinoids

Endocannabinoids are synthesized on demand within the postsynaptic nerve part. This is in contrast with other neurotransmitters which are stored in small vesicles (bubbles) in the presynaptic part of the nerve endings. Once endocannabinoids are released from the plasma membrane of the postsynaptic part of synapse, they travel in a retrograde (backwards) direction across the synaptic gap between two nerves. They then bind to the receptors and temporarily influence presynaptic neurotransmitter release.[195] In this case, the CB receptors are located pre-synaptically.

To date, at least six endocannabinoids have been identified: anandamide, 2-AG, 2-Arachidonyl glyceryl ether, N-Arachidonoyl dopamine, Virodhamine, and Lysophosphatidylinositol.[196]

The two best-characterized endocannabinoids to date are anandamide and 2-AG.[197] The endogenous (internally created) cannabinoid anandamide was discovered in 1992 while 2-AG was first described in 1995.[198,199]

Anandamide (the so-called "bliss" hormone[200]) binds to CB1 receptors but has a very weak affinity for CB2 receptors. Affinity in this case defines the strength of the binding to a receptor. 2-AG on the other hand has a higher affinity to both CB1 and CB2 receptors.

Research showed that anandamide especially can act on other receptors besides CB1 and CB2. This enables anandamide to work in a variety of ways to support the homeostasis of our body.[201] This can be shown with certain conditions of the brain.

Research indicates that anandamide may be part of a natural compensatory mechanism for psychosis in the brain, in the sense that it is elevated in response to onset of psychosis, and the degree of elevation determines the degree of antipsychotic buffering.[202] It was therefore suggested that anandamide elevation in acute paranoid schizophrenia may reflect a compensatory adaptation to the disease,[203] confirming again the concept of homeostasis produced by our own endocannabinoids.

Anandamide is degraded with the help of fatty acid amide hydrolase (FAAH). So, when the enzyme FAAH is inhibited, more anandamide is available to exert its action. We now know that CBD doesn't just bind directly to CB receptors, but also inhibits FAAH and therefore increases internal anandamide levels.[204,205]

In fact, many scientists currently think that this effect is more important than the CB receptor binding. To make things a little more complicated, we now also know that certain proteins, fatty acid-binding proteins (FABPs), inhibit anandamide transport to its destruction enzyme FAAH, which again results in higher anandamide levels.[206] These FABPs are also activated by CBD.

Therefore, the current scientific knowledge surrounding CBD nicely demonstrates that a human body has multiple ways through which CBD can increase the levels of anandamide, supporting many benefits in our body.

Elevated anandamide levels resulting from intake of CBD promote neuroprotective,[207] cardioprotective,[208] anticancer,[209] immune stimulating,[210] and anti-inflammatory effects[211]. Anandamide was also found to be important for gut function,[212,213] pain modulation,[214] uterine-embryo interaction,[215] gastrointestinal as well as urogenital tract function (acting as a spasmolytic),[216,217] maintenance of bone mass,[218] and eye health.[219]

Anandamide often acts as a partial agonist (a substance which initiates a physiological response when combined with a receptor) at CB receptors whereas 2-AG acts as a full agonist in most cases.[220] This suggests that 2-AG has a stronger effect at some of these receptors compared to anandamide.

Recent research showed that 2-AG has an important role in synaptic plasticity (the first stage of rewiring the brain and creating new brain pathways), sensation, and behavioral responses.

In addition, 2-AG was found to be involved in regulation of food intake,[221] obesity,[222] anxiety, pain, stress and fear responses, social behavior,[223] and movement disorders. 2-AG was found to be elevated in brain and nerve conditions such as ischemia (lack of blood flow) and stroke,[224] traumatic brain injury, Parkinson's disease,[225] and multiple sclerosis,[226] indicating a possible role for 2-AG under these conditions.[227]

2-AG has been found present in the brain at concentrations 170 times greater than anandamide.[228] We now know that 2-AG is involved in the synaptic regulation of γ-aminobutyric acid (GABA) and glutamate release, two well-known neurotransmitters.[229] 2-AG is rapidly hydrolyzed (metabolized) by mono-acylglycerol lipase (MAGL) and other enzymes.[230]

Both 2-AG and anandamide are retrograde messengers which means they are released post-synaptically and act pre-synaptically to inhibit release of many excitatory and inhibitory neurotransmitters, including dopamine, glutamate, and GABA.[231]

In conclusion, they both play a very important role in the homeostasis of many different bodily functions and are also influenced positively by the consumption of CBD. It is another beautiful example of how the cells of plants and humans can collaborate in significant ways.

Phytocannabinoids

As a reminder, phytocannabinoids are plant-created. To date, between 100 and 200 phytocannabinoids have been identified. Besides Tetrahydrocannabinol (THC) and Cannabidiol (CBD), the most well-known ones are

Tetrahydrocannabinolic Acid (THCA), Cannabinol (CBN), Cannabigerol (CBG), Cannabidiolic Acid (CBDA), Cannabichromene (CBC), and Tetrahydrocannabivarin (THCV).

I am sure that by the time you read this book, scientists will have found others as this field of research is very much ongoing. At least seven of those phytocannabinoids have been classified as CBD-type compounds including CBD. All of them have the same basic configuration as CBD and vary slightly in the chemical groups attached to the common scaffold. They include CBD, CBDA, CBDVA-C3, CBD-C1, CBD-C4, CBDV, CBDM.[232]

CBD is the main non-psychoactive phytocannabinoid and has little affinity for CB1 and CB2 receptors. As mentioned earlier, CBD inhibits FAAH and therefore increases available anandamide,[233] inhibits release of proinflammatory compounds,[234] activates fatty acid-binding proteins (FABPs) resulting in increased anandamide levels,[235] and acts as an antioxidant and free radical scavenger that is more potent than Vitamin C or Vitamin E.[236]

Most have been under the impression that CBD attaches to mostly CB2 receptors and works that way. However, instead of being a weak agonist, eliciting the same response as other ligands that bind to CB2 receptors, CBD might also have an antagonistic (opposite) effect like blocking the CB2 receptors, highlighting its regulatory potential regarding homeostasis.[237]

Another way for CBD to influence our body is through natural ingredients like β-caryophyllene, which can also be found in Copaiba and many other plants. Other natural compounds like rutamarin from the medicinal plant *Ruta graveolens L.* and 3,3′-diindolylmethane (DIM) from cruciferous vegetables such as broccoli, cauliflower, and kale are also known to bind weakly to CB2 receptors.[238,239] This again highlights the fact that plants, humans, and animals were created in a way to interact and work together.

So, you know that CBD mostly works by influencing the availability of anandamide via manipulating the enzymes needed to break down this endocannabinoid. In addition, it binds weakly to CB1 and CB2 receptors as an agonist but can also function as a potent antagonist on CB2 receptors. So how could it be that CBD works in various, potentially even opposing ways, on CB receptors?

I think we have yet to fully understand how CBD exactly works. But it is generally accepted in science that one of the main functions of CBD is to bring homeostasis to a variety of organ systems. In order to be able to do that, CBD must be able to work through a variety of mechanisms, sometimes supporting and sometimes inhibiting certain reactions in the body. The mechanism constantly changes according to the situation, explaining why it is so difficult to nail down the exact way CBD works. Time will tell if this hypothesis is correct.

Synthetic cannabinoids

Synthetic cannabinoids are created in a lab. Scientists started working with them in the 1970s and at that time they were made of chemical structures derived from THC. Over time, more chemical compounds were developed and selected if they showed affinity to receptors. While THC is only a partial agonist and CBD only a weak agonist, those synthetic analogs sometimes showed extreme high capability to bind to mostly CB1 receptors.

The scary news is that synthetic cannabinoids are being used to enhance regular *Cannabis* plant products. Since the early 90s, literally hundreds of new synthetic compounds have been developed by the pharmaceutical industry. The idea was noble, namely finding alternatives to pain drugs like opioids riddled with side effects and leading to high mortality rates. However, due to their synthetic nature and high affinity to CB receptors, synthetic cannabinoids can be dangerous. Researchers found that some marijuana strains such as "Spice" or "K2" had been sprayed with synthetic cannabinoids to increase their effects.[240]

Synthetic cannabinoids are illegal, except for approved drugs, and are classified as Schedule I. However, some manufacturers have attempted to circumvent these laws by altering the more structurally diverse cannabimimetic compounds in their blends, which might not be listed under scheduled drug regulations.[241]

Synthetic cannabinoids are falsely marketed as safe marijuana substitutes. Many of these dangerous substitutes are easily synthesized, come from China, and are flooding the markets around the world. But it is known that they produce very dangerous adverse effects due to, as of yet, unknown mechanisms. Intoxication with these products can be fatal.[242,243]

A case report about 11 patients intoxicated with synthetic cannabinoids showed that the side effects were altered level of consciousness, severe agitation, seizures, and death.[244] Other authors reported severe hyperthermia (potentially fatal elevation of body temperature) with severe rhabdomyolysis (destruction of muscle tissue leading typically to kidney failure) as well as psychosis.[245,246]

Synthetic cannabinoids such as **AB-PINACA** and **AB-FUBINACA**, sold under the street names Cloud 9, Hookah Relax, Bizarro, Crown, Shisha, Mad Hatter, Bomb Marley, WTF, Diablo, Sexy Monkey, and others, are popular products among young vapers.[247] Strong effects can be achieved with relatively low doses, increasing the risk of intoxication and dangerous side effects.

A report from Turkey revealed that the most common physical symptoms after consumption of a synthetic cannabinoid called Bonzai are eye redness, nausea and vomiting, sweating, and altered mental status including agitation, anxiety, hallucinations, and perceptual changes. Half of the adolescent patients experienced low blood pressure and 31% low heart rate. 25% of the patients had to be transferred to an intensive care unit.[248]

This so-called cannavaping is dangerous when the exact source and contents of the vaped material are not known. It is also not very reassuring that 9 out of 10 cannabinoid vapes contain synthetic cannabinoids as recently reported during a conference.

Cannabinoid Enzymes

The production and the amount of our endocannabinoids anandamide and 2-AG are controlled through a variety of enzymes. The construction crew (a certain set of enzymes) will help to create anandamide and 2-AG while the demolition crew (another set of enzymes) will help to break down anandamide and 2-AG when necessary.

The construction crew/primary biosynthetic enzymes have complicated names like N-acyl-phosphatidylethanolamine-specific phospholipase D (NAPE-PLD) for anandamide[249] and diacylglycerol lipases (DAGL) for 2-AG.[250].

The demolition crew/hydrolytic enzymes are fatty acid amide hydrolase (FAAH) for anandamide and monoacylglycerol lipase (MAGL) and, to a lesser extent, α,β-hydrolase-6 (ABHD-6), cyclooxygenase 2 (COX2), and FAAH1 for 2-AG.

This all sounds very complicated, but I mention these facts not only for those interested in knowing more science, but also because these enzymes can be influenced by other plants.

Examples include the isoflavonoids genistein (found in fava beans, soybeans, kudzu) and daidzein (found in soybeans and other legumes) as well as the flavonoid kaempferol (found in fruits such as apples, grapes, peaches, blackberries, and raspberries, and vegetables such as tomatoes, potatoes, onions, broccoli, lettuce, and spinach).[251,252] The inhibition of these breakdown enzymes opens new ways to increase the action of the endocannabinoids created in our body.[253]

Endocannabinoid Transporters

Most neurotransmitters are water-soluble and easily pass through the watery environment of a synaptic gap. However, our endocannabinoids, like anandamide and 2-AG, are non-charged lipids. Since they are produced in the post-synaptic part of the synapse and must travel backwards across the watery synaptic cleft, they need help. Hence the existence of endocannabinoid transporters, proteins that attach to anandamide and 2-AG to aid them across the gap.

There is also evidence that cholesterol is needed to support the transport of anandamide. One study found that cholesterol could be an important component of the anandamide transport machinery.[254] So lowering cholesterol through statins to very low levels might have an impact on your endocannabinoid system.

One group of scientists found that 2-AG was reduced in patients with heart disease, Type II diabetes, those taking NSAIDs, statins, and anti-diabetic medication.[255] Several other proteins such as fatty-acid-binding proteins, heat shock protein 70, and possibly a fatty acid amide hydrolase-like anandamide transporter protein have been identified to support the transport of endocannabinoids.[256]

Take Away Message
- The endocannabinoid system (ECS) is composed of receptors, ligands, enzymes, and transporters, and its main purpose is to protect multiple organ systems and to keep them in homeostasis.
- Cannabinoid receptors can be found all over the human body. Of the many receptors involved in the

ECS, the most abundant are G-protein receptors known as CB1 and CB2.

- CB1 and CB2 cannabinoid receptors are mostly located in different parts of our body and work through different mechanisms.
- G-protein-coupled receptors are a class of receptors that have an "inbox" on the surface of a cell.
- Receptors can be very specific, meaning that only a certain substance, or ligand, can attach to the receptor. The creation (expression) and removal (degradation) of receptors is in constant flux.
- Binding to CB receptors cause either an increase or a decrease of neurotransmitters released into the synaptic gap.
- As a result, certain reactions in the body can be activated or inhibited.
- If the receptor is a keyhole, a ligand is the key.
- Endocannabinoids are produced within the human body, phytocannabinoids are produced in plants, and synthetic cannabinoids are produced in a lab.
- To date, at least six endocannabinoids have been identified.
- Anandamide (the so-called "bliss" hormone) binds to CB1 receptors but has a very weak affinity for CB2 receptors.
- A human body has multiple ways through which CBD can increase the levels of anandamide, supporting many benefits in our body.
- Anandamide often acts as a partial agonist at CB receptors whereas 2-AG acts as a full agonist in most cases.
- 2-AG has higher affinity to both CB1 and CB2 receptors.
- To date, between 100 and 200 phytocannabinoids have been identified.

- CBD is the main non-psychoactive phytocannabinoid and has little affinity for CB1 and CB2 receptors.
- Another way for CBD to influence our body is through natural ingredients like β-caryophyllene, which can also be found in many other plants.
- Synthetic cannabinoids can be dangerous.
- The production and the amount of anandamide and 2-AG are controlled through a variety of enzymes.
- Endocannabinoid transporters are proteins that attach to anandamide and 2-AG to aid them across the synaptic gap.

Natural Ways to Influence the ECS

Avoidance of toxins

We all know how bad fertilizers, herbicides, and pesticides are for our health. They are even called endocrine disruptors because they influence estrogen receptors in our body and wreak havoc on our endocrine system. My first book describes this problem in detail. These so-called xeno-estrogens (xeno is the old Greek word for foreign) can also bind to CB receptors and block them.[257,258] So avoiding toxic products and embracing a healthy lifestyle will support your ECS and therefore your homeostasis.

Omega fatty acids

Many studies have highlighted the importance of omega-3 fatty acids in regards to the endocannabinoid system.[259] Polyunsaturated fatty acids (PUFA), like omega-3 fatty acids, have shown to be important for neuroprotection, synaptogenesis, and synaptic plasticity.[260] Synaptogenesis is the creation of new connections between nerves, and synaptic plasticity describes the ability of the brain to create new pathways into areas with high synaptic activity.

Arachidonic acid (AA) is an omega-6 PUFA and is among the fatty acids we consume. We need AA for proper functioning of several processes in our body including the biosynthesis of endocannabinoids. Consumption of very high levels of AA leads to inflammation since AA is also broken down into inflammatory compounds. The optimal omega-6 to omega-3 ratio is about three to one, and optimal ratios support health.[261,262] Unfortunately, most people in the civilized world have very high ratios leading to obesity, cardiovascular disease, and other problems.[263,264]

Our own endocannabinoids are also built from AA. However, chronic overconsumption of AA may lead to excessive levels of endocannabinoids which in turn may lead to desensitized and downregulated CB1 and CB2 receptors.[265] Omega-3s on the other hand support greater levels of endocannabinoid synthetic enzymes, increasing anandamide and 2-AG in a balanced way.[266] Consumption of healthy omega-3 fatty acids also modulate the concentrations of other compounds increasing the action of cannabinoids.[267]

Low levels of healthy omega-3 fatty acids are linked to neuropsychiatric diseases. The discovery that fatty acids influence the ECS could explain the behavioral changes caused by omega-3 deficiency that is often observed in western diets.[268] Another study found that the health benefits of omega-3 fatty acids are mediated, in part, through their metabolic conversion to bioactive metabolites of fatty acids. The authors also discovered that plants can contain naturally occurring omega-3–derived cannabinoids and therefore contribute to human health via the ECS.[269]

The omega fatty acid content and ratio that is optimal for human health, as mentioned earlier, is the reason for many of the beneficial effects of dietary hemp seeds.[270] Consumption of hemp seeds has especially shown benefits for the cardiovascular system.[271] Hemp seeds were able to reduce cholesterol-induced blood platelet aggregation (clumping),[272] reducing the risk for cardiovascular pathologies such as stroke or heart attacks.

So, dietary omega-3s seem to act as homeostatic regulators of the ECS. This is just another example how living a healthy lifestyle can influence the endocannabinoid system.

Chocolate

Three substances in chocolate and cocoa powder were found to mimic cannabinoids by activating receptors or increasing anandamide levels.[273] However, it is not certain whether these compounds act by binding directly to CB receptors in the brain or by mostly influencing anandamide levels.[274] Nevertheless, the combination of CBD with chocolate makes sense, not just from a culinary perspective.

Tea

If you like to drink tea, you could also be on your way to supporting your ECS. A study showed that biochanin A found in teas like oolong, but also in foods like red clover, peanuts, and soy is a FAAH inhibitor.[275] Epigallocatechin-3-O-gallate, the most abundant catechin in tea, also has micromolar affinities for CB1.[276] In summary, tea consumption could elevate anandamide levels and support your ECS.

Coffee

Research data demonstrates the ability of caffeine from coffee and other caffeinated beverages to reduce the pathological consequences of stress via supporting CB1 receptors in the brain. Chronic caffeine consumption leads to cannabinoid CB1 receptor stimulation by exo- and endocannabinoids.[277] Exocannabinoids are those coming from plants or synthetic sources, while endocannabinoids such as anandamide and 2-AG are produced within our body as discussed in earlier chapters.

Carrots

Carrots contain a substance called falcarinol, also known as carotatoxin or panaxynol. It is a natural pesticide and fatty alcohol also found in red ginseng, celery, fennel, parsnip, and ivy. Falcarinol demonstrated binding affinity to the two main human CB receptors, CB1 and CB2, and selectively changes the anandamide binding site of CB1 receptors.[278] By doing so it blocks this kind of receptor while still preserving and weakly activating CB2 receptors. In addition, it prevents our own endocannabinoid anandamide from doing its job.

This all sounds negative and in fact, blocking anandamide is not a good thing when it comes to skin allergies. Falcarinol is known to be a skin irritant found in several plants that causes contact dermatitis.[279]

However, it opens the opportunity to block the potentially negative side effects of THC while preserving the beneficial effects of CBD. When would that be important? Maybe when using full-spectrum CBD which likely contains small amounts of THC.

In addition, falcarinol demonstrated cancer cell inhibiting activity.[280] It induces cell death and arrest of the cell cycle, which means that falcarinol makes cancer cells kill themselves and also stops their development during one of the important times of growth.[281] Falcarinol and related compounds also demonstrated anti-inflammatory bioactivity.[282] These are some of the many benefits of eating carrots or similar falcarinol-containing vegetables. When carrots are cooked however, they will lose about 70% of their falcarinol content due to the heat. This is also the reason why carrot seed essential oil does not contain falcarinol.

Yangonin (Kava)

Originally, kava came from Polynesia. Over time, the original plant made its way to other places around the world including New Zealand. There it did not flourish too well and was replaced with another plant that we now call Kava. The original Kava is therefore different from today's Kava. Research found that Kava activates both CB1 and CB2 receptors while not exerting too much influence on the enzyme system used to breakdown endogenous anandamide or 2-AG.[283] Kava binds with higher affinity to CB1 compared to CB2 receptors.[284] This mechanism could explain the anxiolytic (anxiety-reducing) properties of Kava.

Turmeric

Curcumin, extracted from turmeric, elevates endocannabinoid levels and the brain nerve growth factor.[285] It has been suggested that the combined use of marijuana and turmeric is potentially beneficial in gastrointestinal disease.[286] However, the authors warned that more research is needed, especially comparing this combination with standard therapies. Curcumin is also regarded to be an absorption enhancer for cannabinoids such as CBD, increasing its bioavailability.[287,288] The bioavailability of curcumin itself can be increased by 2,000% when piperine from black pepper is added.[289] So the addition of curcumin (and possibly piperine) to CBD is very intriguing.

Wormwood

Another natural substance known to bind to CB1 and CB2 receptors is the terpenoid thujone found in wormwood. As mentioned earlier, wormwood, also called *Artemisia absinthium*, is an ancient herbal medicine primarily used for digestion or to kill worms. Wormwood is used to produce absinthe, an emerald-green liqueur that achieved enormous popularity at the close of the 19th century.

However, thujone by itself is a GABA-A receptor antagonist that can cause convulsions and death when administered in large amounts.[290] The consumption of thujone containing products was outlawed in many countries, partly during the time of alcohol prohibition but also because of its potentially fatal side effects. More recent research however hints to its beneficial effects regarding neuroprotection after a stroke and for patients with Crohn's disease when using it in an appropriate dose.[291]

Sage

Sage, or *Salvia officinalis* L., translates into "medical cure". Salvia stands for rescue or cure while officinalis describes medical use. Sage has been used for centuries as an antiseptic, antiscabies, antisyphilitic, and anti-inflammatory and has frequently be applied against skin and eye diseases, digestive problems, and in pleurisy, an inflammation of the thin skin surrounding the lungs.[292]

Only a few know that sage, and therefore sage essential oil, also contains the monoterpene thujone. In fact, sage essential oil can contain up to 50% thujone and because we typically only use one or two drops of sage at any given time, there are no side effects to be expected. This is confirmed by current regulations regarding the ingestion of thujone-containing products.[293] In addition, the FDA has declared sage to be GRAS (Generally Regarded As Safe).

Because of the structural similarity of thujone enol with THC, it was speculated that plants containing thujone may activate cannabinoid receptors, especially CB1 receptors.[294,295] A group of researchers found that thujone in fact binds weakly to both CB1 and CB2 receptors, but also noted the hypothesis that activation of cannabinoid receptors is responsible for the intoxicating effects of thujone is not supported by the present data.[296]

Sage, and other plants and spices such as clove, basil, spearmint, hops, and ginseng, also contain humulene (α-caryophyllene) which is similar to β-caryophyllene. Humulene has strong anti-inflammatory properties.[297] It also seems to bind to CB2 receptors, although no good article on this subject could yet be found. All in all, the addition of sage to CBD is an interesting concept.

Echinacea

Echinacea, a flowering plant in the daisy family, is also very interesting when it comes to the endocannabinoid system. Echinacea has shown to be effective against the common cold and other respiratory infections.[298] The scientific community has not yet reached an agreement on whether it also effectively fights cancer cells. But one thing is clear, echinacea has affinity to CB1 and CB2 receptors, and it seems that it binds better to CB2 than compared to CB1.[299] In addition, echinacea inhibits the reuptake of anandamide. This means that either more anandamide is available to interact with the endocannabinoid receptors, or that it binds for a longer time to the receptors.

A group of scientists showed that the N-alkylamides from echinacea act via modulation of the endocannabinoid system by simultaneously targeting the CB2 receptor, endocannabinoid transport, and degradation.[300] Overall, the CB2 receptor-binding N-alkylamides show similar anti-inflammatory effects as anandamide itself.[301]

And because the exact mechanism by which echinacea works is still unclear, researchers are starting to think that it might be related to the fact that it binds to CB2 receptors while increasing the activity of our endocannabinoid anandamide.[302] Perhaps this is how echinacea supports the immune system during conditions such as the common flu.

Black Pepper

Black pepper is an interesting plant/spice in the sense that it has multiple effects on the endocannabinoid system. Firstly, *Piper nigrum*, or simply black pepper, contains about 25-35% β-caryophyllene (BCP) which selectively binds to CB2 receptors. BCP is one of the major components found in hemp leaves, but it is not found in hemp stalks. As mentioned earlier, many plants such as copaiba, clove, *Cannabis*, rosemary, oregano, lavender, cinnamon, ylang ylang, basil, and hops contain various amounts of this important sesquiterpene.

Secondly, black pepper also contains a substance called guineensine which has shown to inhibit cellular uptake of anandamide.[303] Guineensine however did not inhibit endocannabinoid degrading enzymes FAAH or monoacylglycerol lipase (MAGL), nor did it interact directly with cannabinoid receptors. This highlights the fact that black pepper influences the endocannabinoid system in a variety of distinct ways. Guineensine also interreacts with other non-CB-related receptors supporting the anti-inflammatory role black pepper can have in our body.[304]

And thirdly, the presence of black pepper has shown to improve absorption of many nutrients. This effect is likely due to a compound called piperine. Dietary piperine, by favorably stimulating the digestive enzymes of the pancreas, enhances the digestive capacity and significantly reduces the gastrointestinal food transit time.[305] By influencing the way the liver breaks down absorbed nutrients and medical drugs, piperine has been documented to enhance the bioavailability of a number of therapeutic drugs as well as phytochemicals.[306]

Black pepper and other types of pepper induce a change in the gut wall, resulting in an increased absorptive surface of the small intestine.[307] It was also suggested that the increased absorption has to do with changes in enzyme activity within the gut wall.[308] And last but not

113

least, piperine has shown to bind to the human vanilloid receptor TRPV1, a receptor to which CBD also binds.[309]

Some authors believe that its anti-inflammatory and anti-cancer effects stem from its multiple ways to influence immune modulation.[310,311] In addition, black pepper is also known to assist in cognitive brain functioning.[312] The metabolites of black pepper are known to improve epilepsy, Parkinson's disease, depression, and pain related disorders.[313]

Other authors have summarized the immunomodulatory, antioxidant, anti-asthmatic, anti-carcinogenic, anti-inflammatory, anti-ulcer, and anti-amoebic properties of black pepper.[314,315] All in all, these properties make black pepper an interesting plant to potentially add to CBD, either ground up or in essential oil form. It should also be noted that black pepper essential oil does not contain piperine or guineensine largely due to poor solubility in steam.

Olive Oil and Other Polyphenols

It is well known that olives and olive-based products contain very beneficial polyphenols and potent antioxidants. Extra virgin cold pressed olive oil has been a main component of the Mediterranean diet, famous for its longevity-promoting effects.[316] Recent studies showed that extra virgin olive oil (EVOO) also influences the endocannabinoid system.

This effect seems to be isolated to influencing genes that promote the upregulation of CB1 receptors. In fact, CB1 expression in the colon increased four-fold after consumption of EVOO.[317] The appearance of CB receptors is not a static thing. CB1 and CB2, as well as other receptors involved in the endocannabinoid system, increase and decrease in numbers as needed.

One mechanism responsible for these changes is the expression of genes, which means that the command contained in the genes is carried out. EVOO is able to get such genes to express which protect the body from inflammation, cardiovascular events, neurological damage, metabolic problems, as well as cancer growth, all of which promote longevity.[318] Other polyphenols such as curcumin and trans-resveratrol have also shown to bind to CB1 receptors and block them.[319]

Flavonoids

Certain flavonoids like genistein and daidzein inhibit FAAH. Genistein is found in fava beans, soybeans, and coffee.[320] Daidzein is a naturally occurring compound found exclusively in soybeans and other legumes[321] Other flavonoids such as biochanin A and kaempferol also exert modest inhibition of FAAH.[322] By doing so, all these healthy plant compounds increase the availability of anandamide and support the ECS.

Other Alternative Methods

Complementary and alternative medicine interventions also upregulate and modulate the ECS system. Such interventions include massage and manipulation, acupuncture, dietary supplements, and herbal medicines as well as lifestyle modifications including diet, weight control, exercise, and the use of psychoactive substances such as alcohol, tobacco, coffee, or marijuana.[323]

Temperature

Cold temperatures are known to increase endocannabinoid levels and to improve the density of CB1 neurons in certain parts of the brain by up to 40%.[324] Cold temperatures increase the endocannabinoid tone.[325] We also know that endocannabinoids participate in the febrile (fever) response.[326] While research revealed that the ECS is part of the thermoregulatory system, no studies could be found explaining how lowering body temperature could benefit humans in regard to the ECS.

Take Away Message
- Avoiding toxic products and embracing a healthy lifestyle will support your ECS and therefore your homeostasis.
- Many studies have highlighted the importance of omega-3 fatty acids to the ECS.
- Substances in chocolate and cocoa powder were found to mimic cannabinoids.
- Tea consumption could elevate anandamide levels.
- Caffeine from coffee can reduce the pathological consequences of stress via supporting CB1 receptors in the brain.
- Carrots contain a substance called falcarinol, which demonstrated binding affinity to CB1 and CB2.
- Curcumin, extracted from turmeric, elevates endocannabinoid levels andis also regarded to be an absorption enhancer for cannabinoids such as CBD.
- Sage has been used for centuries as an antiseptic, antiscabies, antisyphilitic, and anti-inflammatory compound. Sage contains thujone which binds weakly to both CB1 and CB2 receptors.
- Echinacea has affinity to CB1 and CB2 receptors.

- *Piper nigrum*, black pepper, contains about 25-35% β-caryophyllene (BCP). The presence of black pepper has shown to improve absorption of many nutrients.
- Recent studies showed that extra virgin olive oil (EVOO) also positively influences the endocannabinoid system.
- Certain flavonoids found in fava beans, soybeans, and coffee increase the availability of anandamide and support the ECS.
- Cold temperatures are known to increase endocannabinoid levels and improve the density of CB1 neurons in certain parts of the brain by up to 40%.

CBD and the Human Body

Pharmacokinetics of CBD

Pharmacokinetics describes the ways in which drugs move through the body including absorption, distribution, metabolism/breakdown, and excretion. Pharmacodynamics describes what kind of an effect a substance can have in the body. In this chapter we will concentrate on the pharmacokinetics of CBD. This is important because this knowledge will guide you when it comes to selecting a formulation and a route of intake for CBD.

But let's go through this pharmacokinetics thing step-by-step and look at what we know about absorption, distribution, metabolism, and excretion when it comes to CBD. Be aware of the fact that the vast majority of studies looked at the pharmacokinetics of THC and THC containing products and not isolated CBD. Therefore, it is somewhat difficult to find good data on CBD alone.

Absorption

Humans and animals can absorb CBD in a variety of ways involving different organ systems. It can be swallowed (oral application), and then it will go through the gut wall into the blood stream. CBD can be applied into the nose (intra-nasal) and absorb into the blood vessels there. It can be put under the tongue (sublingual) or swished around in the mouth (intra-orally), where the CBD will absorb directly into the oral blood vessels. When we then swallow, whatever is left will go through the gut wall. CBD can be applied topically to the skin and absorb into the body that way (transdermal application). It can also be applied rectally (rectal application) and absorb into the blood vessels of the rectum.

CBD can be breathed in (via inhaling, smoking, or vaporizing) and absorb into the blood vessels of the lungs. It can be applied to the eyes with eyedrops (ophthalmic application). CBD can even be taken intravenously in which case no absorption is necessary since it is added directly into the blood. And in animal research it is also injected intraperitoneally (IP administration) which means that it is injected into the space in the abdomen surrounding the gut because this space has many blood vessels.

As mentioned above, when you swallow your CBD in the form of edibles, tea, oils, or some other option, it will go through the gut wall into the blood vessels of the gut and then pass through the liver before it continues its travel through the body. Oral CBD undergoes extensive first-pass metabolism in the liver via the enzyme Cytochrome P450 3A4 (CYP3A4), with a relatively low bioavailability of 6-30%.[327] CYP3A4 belongs to a group of important enzymes called the cytochrome P450 system, mainly found in the liver and in the intestine but also in other places such as lungs, kidneys, and blood.[328]

These types of enzymes help the body to remove certain toxins and drugs and also some plant compounds such as CBD. All of this has two consequences when looking at CBD. Much of the CBD will be broken down/metabolized before it can even reach other parts of the body, and, because CBD is broken down by CYP enzymes, it will interfere with the breakdown of other substances such as medical drugs. It is well known that CBD is a major and potent inhibitor of P450-mediated hepatic drug metabolism.[329,330] But CBD also inhibits other CYP enzymes in the liver.[331,332,333]

Since it is almost completely absorbed by the gut wall, oral application and swallowing of CBD has a very low bioavailability. Luckily, we can add other compounds to CBD such as oil (hemp oil, olive oil, or avocado oil for example), ground black pepper, and/or curcumin, or choose a different application method to increase absorption and/or bioavailability.

All other routes of administrations besides oral tend to avoid the first-pass effect in the liver and therefore increase bioavailability, provided that the absorption is good. Absorption through the skin can be tricky and low depending on the type of formulation used. So, even if the CBD then avoids the first-pass effect, the overall bioavailability can still be low because so little CBD makes it through the skin.

Again, specific formulations can substantially enhance the absorption though the skin. Most common forms of intake of CBD are oral, sublingual/intra-oral, and topical/transdermal. All other ways to take CBD are either for research purposes or when taking CBD as part of THC, like smoking pot.

As mentioned earlier, studies have shown that the bioavailability of orally ingested CBD is around 6%. When inhaled via smoking, the bioavailability of CBD was measured at around 31%.[334] Other studies reported it to be as high as 56% when consumed via the lungs.[335]

The same group of scientists also mentioned that the absorption through the gut wall can be increased when combining CBD with other substance such as olive oil, sesame oil, or turmeric. Most of that CBD will still be immediately metabolized by the liver, but because more CBD goes to the liver there is a good chance that more will be available after passing through it.

Researchers also found other reasons for low bioavailability such as variable absorption in the gut, depending on whether cannabinoids were taken on an empty stomach or not, degradation of cannabinoids in the stomach, interaction with other cannabinoids, as well as the formation of inactive metabolites in the liver.[336,337]

Distribution

Data on how exactly CBD is distributed within the body seems to be lacking. However, one study revealed that in five autopsy cases, distribution of cannabinoids showed relatively high CBD concentrations in bile and muscle tissues. It was noted that the CBD content of the brain was unexpectedly high.[338] Another study looking at CBD distribution in the brain found equal distribution throughout all brain regions.[339]

Metabolism

Metabolism refers to the breakdown of a substance. CBD undergoes extensive metabolism at multiple sites.[340] As mentioned earlier, the liver with its CYP enzymes is one of the main places in the body where CBD is metabolized. Altogether, some 100 CBD metabolites have been identified.

Excretion/Elimination

CBD is either excreted intact or in the form of one of its metabolites.[341] More than 40 metabolites have been identified in excretion products such as urine or bile.[342] O-glucuronide conjugate of CBD was one of the most abundant urinary excretion products (13.3%), while the concentration of intact urinary CBD was 12.1%.

The half-life (the period of time required for the concentration or amount of drug in the body to be reduced by one-half) of CBD in humans was found to be between 18 to 33 hours following intravenous administration, 27 to 35 hours following smoking, one to two days when taken orally in single doses, and two to five days following repeated oral administration.[343,344,345,346]

CBD and the Brain

The brain is made up of different cells. Two of the main categories include neural cells, those that process information and then pass it on to the next cell(s), and non-neural cells. The non-neural cells are also called the glial cells. The human brain contains an estimated 100 billion neural cells and around 85 billion glia-type cells. Some call the collection of glial cells the glia brain. Glial cells have five main functions:[347]

> (1) to surround neurons and hold them in place like glue, so they are sometimes called the glue of the brain. In fact, the word glia comes from the Ancient Greek word for glue
>
> (2) to supply nutrients and oxygen to neurons
>
> (3) to insulate one neuron from another

(4) to destroy pathogens and remove dead neurons, so they are sometimes called the janitors of the brain

(5) to support neurotransmission and help create new synaptic connections.

Glial cells include oligodendrocytes, astrocytes, ependymal cells, and microglia. In the peripheral nervous system, glial cells include Schwann cells and satellite cells. The most abundant form of glial cells are astrocytes. These astrocytes are involved in the formation of the blood-brain-barrier, in the blood supply of the neurons, as well as in the regulation and recycling of neurotransmitters. Neurons express mostly CB1 cannabinoid receptors, while glial cells express CB2.

Interestingly, both types of the cannabinoid receptors were found to be present on astrocytes.[348] This is a clear indication that cannabinoids, whether they are produced within the body in the form of endocannabinoids or consumed from plants as phytocannabinoids, have an important role in brain function and brain homeostasis.

The brain protects itself from being invaded by toxins present in the blood by creating and maintaining the blood-brain-barrier. Astrocytes are involved in the creation of this isolation between blood vessels and brain tissue. CBD preserves the functionality of the blood-brain-barrier after oxygen deprivation, as seen after a stroke. It does this via activation of different types of receptors other than CB receptors.[349] After a stroke, the concentration of endocannabinoids and the number of CB receptors in the brain are increased to promote neuroprotection.[350] These findings again highlight the potential for compounds like CBD to protect the brain from damage and support its recovery.

I mentioned earlier that CBD has shown to have weak affinity (binding capacity) to CB receptors in the brain. The evidence is mounting that CBD does not influence brain function by direct binding to CB receptors, but rather works by influencing some of the enzymes used in the ECS. This increases the availability of anandamide which then influences brain function. Simply expressed, CBD is more like the police officer directing traffic rather than the driver of a car.

We also know from recent research that CBD affects synaptic plasticity and facilitates neurogenesis (the formation of new brain neurons).[351] So endocannabinoids have emerged as mediators of short- and long-term synaptic plasticity in diverse brain structures.[352]

The term synaptic plasticity describes the ability of the brain to start forming new synapses or in other words, enable the brain to create new and more connections between nerves or brain cells during the process of learning or changing habits.[353] It is well known today that synaptic plasticity is necessary for learning and memorizing new things or forming new habits.[354]

Short-term plasticity describes the mechanism by which special adjacent brain nerves, known as neurons, "stretch" themselves into an area of higher activity to see what is going on. We call this process neuronal sprouting.[355] Higher activity is usually defined as the occurrence of increased electrical activity or the production and release of more neurotransmitters.

As the process evolves, the glial cells get involved. The interaction of neurons with higher activity during learning and glial cells which sprout in these areas of higher activity to see what is going on eventually creates new brain pathways. The initial glial-neuronal interactions contribute to short-term synaptic plasticity and short-term memory. Glial cells have been reported to modulate synaptic plasticity in many ways.[356]

The fact that some of these glial cells contain CB receptors highlights the importance of the ECS in the formation of new brain pathways. In fact, recent research specifically shows that CBD stimulated neurogenesis and promoted brain nerve restructuring in certain areas after damage due to lack of oxygen. The authors concluded that short-term CBD treatment results in global functional recovery during and after ischemic (lack of blood flow) brain injury and impacts multiple and distinct targets involved in the pathophysiology of brain ischemic injury.[357]

Long-term plasticity describes the establishment of new synaptic connections between nerves, hence supporting long-term memory and new brain pathways.[358] This entire process is then called neuroplasticity. Neuroplasticity describes the brain's capability to rewire itself.

And because you now know that CBD is involved in synaptic plasticity and neuroplasticity and therefore in the formation of memories related to emotions, it becomes clear that the endocannabinoid system plays a critical role in the regulation of emotions. Understanding how CBD regulates emotion and emotional memory processing will eventually lead to its use as an established treatment for anxiety-related and substance abuse disorders.[359]

Because changes in the endocannabinoid system may be an important factor in the etiology/origination of neuropsychiatric disorders, phytocannabinoids like CBD play a role in the prevention and treatment of such conditions. Enhancers of endocannabinoid signaling could represent a potential therapeutic tool in the treatment of mood swings, anxiety, and depression.[360]

New evidence also indicates that CBD is able to reduce fear in different ways[361]:

(1) by decreasing acute fear
(2) by reducing fear upon fearful memory retrieval
(3) by enhancing extinction of fear
(4) by reducing fear connected to specific noises.

This why CBD is currently being evaluated for anxiety and fear disorders, PTSD, and other related conditions.

All these findings and evidence highlight the important role of the endocannabinoid system, and potentially CBD, in improved functioning of the brain as well as in emotional homeostasis.[362]

Do the Bugs in Your Gut Care About CBD?

What is the microbiome? By definition it is the collective genome (genetic information) of all your micro-organisms such as bacteria, fungi, viruses, and archaea (bacteria-like organisms).[363] You harbor over 100 trillion of them, and most of them can be found in your gut, mainly the colon.[364]

Bacteria from various microbiome systems interact extensively with each other within the human body.[365] The microbiome has also been called "the last undiscovered human organ" highlighting the importance it has in human health.[366] It might be a little scary for you to hear this, but your microbiome cells outnumber your human cells by 10 to one.[367]

And if you look at the genetic information contained in the microbiome, the news gets even worse. It is estimated that 99% of the genetic information in a human body comes from the microbes and only roughly 1% is part of your own genetic information contained in the DNA obtained from your parents.[368]

Researchers found that the microbiome contains 150 times more individual genes than human DNA, namely 3.3 million different genes compared to "only" 23,000 human genes.[369,370] The diversity among the microbiome of individuals is immense: individual humans are about 99.9% identical to one another in terms of genetic information contained in the DNA but can be 80-90% different from one another in terms of the genetic information contained in the microbiome of their gut and skin.[371]

Why would there be a connection between the gut, microbiome, endocannabinoid system, and CBD? We know that glial cells contain CB receptors. We also know that the gut is rich in CB2 receptors and contains CB1 receptors. Also, the gut has its own nervous system called the enteric nervous system which contains glial cells too. In fact, they are called enteric glial cells, and they actively control acute and chronic inflammation in the gut.[372] Are you starting to connect the dots?

Evidence has accumulated in recent years that cannabinoids inhibit gastric and intestinal motility through activation of enteric CB1 receptors.[373] CB1 receptors have also be found to be involved in the control of gastroesophageal reflux and nausea and vomiting.[374] Activation of CB2 receptors in the enteric nervous system was able to dampen endotoxin-induced enhanced intestinal contractility and therefore reduce gut spasms and normalize bowel movements.[375,376]

Gut motility also has an influence on the microbiome. In fact, it is one of the ways that the brain can control and influence bacterial composition in the gut. By sending signals via the vagal nerve to the gut, the brain effects the enteric nervous system and bowel movement activity which in turn can influence the composition of the microbiome.

One scientific review clearly states that gut microorganisms, i.e. the microbiome, and the endocannabinoid system are intertwined.[377] The authors of this review paper also mention that the ECS is involved in numerous biological processes including control of gut inflammation and gut-barrier function.

They also connect an altered ECS to obesity, diabetes, and metabolic syndrome which all contribute to the onset of cardiometabolic diseases. During the past decade, it became clear that the composition of the microbes in the gut plays an important role in the regulation of body weight and therefore in the pathophysiology of obesity. It is especially clear that the type of food ingested will directly influence the microbiome.[378,379]

More recent research now connects the quality of the microbiome to the presence of the ECS. Inflammation in the gut releases inflammatory compounds such as lipopolysaccharide (LPS) which is an endotoxin released by bad bacteria. Blockage or inactivation of CB receptors resulted in an increase of LPS, compromising gut wall integrity. Both, changes in the composition of the microbiome and tone of the ECS, resulted in increased adipogenesis (formation of body fat).

One study described that the gut microbiome modulates the intestinal ECS tone, which in turn regulates gut wall permeability and LPS levels.[380] Endocannabinoid signaling mechanisms in the gut have been suggested to play an important role in the control of food intake and energy balance.[381]

This all shows that your lifestyle, food intake, physical activity, gut, microbiome, brain, and ECS are completely connected and any disturbance will have health consequences. The connections relating to the ECS have been named the gut-microbiota-endocannabinoid system axis. We also know that the gut has many CB2 receptors and that CBD will likely have a positive effect on your gut.[382] This is why studies show good results when treating intestinal inflammation[383], irritable or inflammatory bowel syndrome[384,385], bowel colic, and colitis with CBD and/or THC.

It is also well established that THC-containing products can be used to reduce nausea and vomiting.[386] In fact, one of the first recognized medical uses of THC was treatment of chemotherapy-induced nausea and vomiting.[387] What is not well known is the fact that both CB1 and CB2 receptors are involved in the control of emesis (vomiting). Blocking CB1 receptors resulted in nausea, while activation of CB1 and CB2 receptors via internal (endocannabinoids) and external (phytocannabinoids) cannabinoids both resulted in reduced nausea and vomiting.[388] Interestingly, the endocannabinoids involved in improving nausea are not as much related to anandamide as they are to 2-AG.[389]

It also important to mention that the microbes of the gut microbiome regulate the expression of receptors such as 5-HT1A and others in the brain and elsewhere.[390] The intake of probiotics may help control the PPARγ receptor, the "master regulator" of adipogenesis (formation of fat), and TNF-α, an inflammation marker.[391] The fact that CBD influences receptors like CB1, CB2, 5-HT1A, and PPARγ just underlines the importance that it can have in the regulation of the microbiome. Also, probiotics and prebiotics both modulate CB1 expression.[392]

You can now start to see how all dots connect: your gut, diet, lifestyle, microbiome, brain, memory, emotions, immune system, ECS, and cannabinoids. No wonder that CBD is seen by many as a miracle even if they do not understand all of these connections.

CBD and Hormones

In general, there is very little scientific data regarding hormonal changes in humans when consuming CBD. A few studies looked mainly at the effects of THC. You probably know by now that CBD has a relaxing effect. This stress-reducing effect is part of the function of the ECS in our body.

And whenever stress reduces, the stress hormone cortisol likely also reduces. That was shown in a study investigating several hormone levels after consumption of CBD. The authors of that study concluded that CBD reduces cortisol.[393]

One animal study suggested that raw marijuana extracts decreased sex hormone levels like testosterone. It was however unclear whether this was caused by THCa, CBDa, or any other compound found in marijuana.[394] THCa and CBDa are the raw acidic precursors of THC and CBD. Another study looked at inhaled and ingested THC and found it depressed testosterone by 20-30% and thyroid hormone triiodothyronine (T3) by 17-29%.[395] Again, these changes seem to be specific to THC and not CBD.

One study compared THC and CBD in acute and chronic application and found that both THC and CBD decreased testosterone when given short-term, but only THC and not CBD decreased testosterone when given long-term.[396] Changes in sex hormone levels seem to be related to the enzymes needed to break down marijuana, as this breakdown mechanism competes with the metabolism of other medications or in this case hormones.

Excess food intake and obesity enhance the ECS tone which leads this delicate system into overdrive. A hyperactive ECS contributes to visceral fat accumulation and obesity by reducing energy expenditure and by enhancing both food intake and lipogenesis.[397] THC increases appetite but the effect of CBD on appetite seems somewhat controversial. I always advise combining a healthier food intake, physical exercise, and CBD to rebalance the ECS.

One study investigated the effects of CBD on a variety of metabolism markers and found that it decreased resistin, a hormone that was recently identified and links obesity to Type 2 diabetes, and increased glucose-dependent insulinotropic peptide.[398] The main function of glucose-dependent insulinotropic peptide is to stimulate insulin secretion in order to lower blood sugar.

High resistin levels lead to insulin resistance, diabetes, atherosclerosis, cardiovascular disease, non-alcoholic fatty liver disease, autoimmune disease, malignancy, asthma, inflammatory bowel disease, and chronic kidney disease.[399] Therefore, the resistin-lowering effect of CBD is good for overall health.

CBD and Physical Activity

Acute aerobic exercise improves mood and activates the ECS in physically active individuals.[400] But most studies on athletic performance researched the effects of marijuana/THC on athletes and not the effects of CBD. One review of medical literature found that there is no direct evidence of performance-enhancing effects of cannabinoids in athletes. However, they mentioned the beneficial effects of marijuana as part of pain management and reduction of concussion-related symptoms.[401]

Another review of 15 studies evaluated athletic performance connected to the effects of THC in association with exercise protocols. Of these studies, none showed any improvement in aerobic performance.[402]

We know that CBD supports elevated levels of anandamide, and that could be one of the mechanisms through which athletes could benefit from CBD. Researchers found that humans and dogs share significantly increased exercise-induced endocannabinoid signaling following high-intensity endurance running. However, endocannabinoid signaling does not significantly increase following low-intensity walking.[403] They concluded that exercise results in positive neurological changes and that the so-called "runners high" may also be linked to the ECS.

Another study measured endocannabinoid levels in treadmill users running at four different intensity levels. The results showed significantly increased endocannabinoid levels following moderate intensities only, whereas very high as well as very low intensity exercises did not significantly alter circulating endocannabinoid levels. So, endocannabinoid signaling is indeed intensity dependent and is optimal in moderate exercise.[404]

Anandamide, when available in a sufficient dose, can improve muscle glucose uptake and activate some key molecules of insulin signaling and mitochondrial biogenesis. More mitochondria mean more energy. These effects probably happen because anandamide interacts at receptors which may trigger positive metabolic effects. Consumption of CBD with subsequent elevated anandamide levels could be an important factor in optimizing energy levels for an active lifestyle.

133

Exercise indeed increased endocannabinoid levels, even in patients with major depressive disorders.[405] It was concluded that exercise is a good therapeutic modality for such patients. CBD consumption alone is also beneficial in depressive disorders.[406,407] Therefore, one could argue that the combination of CBD consumption and exercise should be recommended for depressive and anxious patients.

One study revealed that aerobic exercise significantly reduced the CB1 receptor expression in certain areas of the brain, including the hippocampus.[408] The same was shown by another group of scientists who investigated the relationship between CB1 receptors, obesity, and weight loss (measured by reduction of fat cells) through exercise.[409] Since CB1 expression is elevated in obese patients, a reduction of CB1 receptors, especially in fat cells, in this population is a good thing. The authors concluded that the connection between exercise and the amount of CB1 receptors is important for the reduction of fat tissue.

CBD and Body Weight/Obesity (Why Your Fat Cells Care)

Obesity may be seen as a modern weapon of mass destruction. It reached levels of a global epidemic.[410] In most countries, women have higher obesity rates than men. And obesity is usually now associated with poverty, even in developing countries.[411] Overall, obesity is fueled by economic growth, industrialization, mechanized transport, urbanization, an increasingly sedentary lifestyle, and a nutritional transition to processed foods and high calorie diets over the last 30 years.[412]

In that time frame, many countries have witnessed the prevalence of obesity in its citizens double and even quadruple. Prevalence is the proportion of a population who have a specific characteristic in a given time period.[413] After remaining relatively stable in the 1960s and 1970s, the prevalence of obesity among adults in the United States increased by approximately 50% per decade throughout the 1980s and 1990s.[414] About a third of today's world population is currently obese.[415]

In the U.S., the direst projections based on earlier trends point to over 85% of adults being overweight or obese by 2030. In addition, by 2048, all American adults would become overweight or obese, while African-American women will reach that state by 2034 if the current trend continues. In children, the prevalence of obesity will nearly double by 2030.

Total health-care costs attributable to obesity and excessive weight would double every decade to 957 billion U.S. dollars by 2030, accounting for 16-18% of total U.S. health-care costs.[416] Luckily, in recent years, national estimates of obesity seem to indicate that the steady upward trend of obesity in Americans over the past three to five decades has leveled off at a prevalence of about 35%.[417]

However, this is no reason to celebrate. Researchers estimate that the overall negative effect of obesity on life expectancy in the United States is a reduction of one third to three fourths of a year. This reduction in life expectancy is not trivial. It is larger than the negative effects of all accidental deaths such as accidents, homicides, and suicides combined.[418] And the reduction in life expectancy is expected to grow to two to five years in the coming decades. This is the first time in the history of mankind that researchers predict that our children will not live as long as we do! This is a very sad finding.

Our endocannabinoid system was identified to include a group of molecules that significantly contributes to metabolic control and therefore weight control.[419] In fact, our endocannabinoids anandamide and 2-AG are deeply involved in all aspects of the control of energy balance.

Early in life, activation of CB1 receptors seems to be involved in suckling.[420] The authors of that study concluded that the endocannabinoid system plays a vital role in milk suckling, and hence in growth and development during the early stages of life, at least in mice. It is very interesting that anandamide-treated mice during lactation showed a significant increase in accumulated food intake, body weight, and epididymal fat (some of the fat in the belly) during adulthood when compared to control mice.

When evaluating CB1 receptor occurrence in epididymal fat, the anandamide-treated group showed a 150% increase in expression. This group also displayed significantly higher levels of circulating glucose, insulin, leptin, triglycerides, cholesterol, and NEFA. In addition, significant levels of insulin resistance were another important finding in the anandamide-treated group.[421] The same group of scientists concluded that progressive increase in body fat accumulation can be programmed in early stages of life by oral treatment with the endocannabinoid anandamide.[422]

This does not mean that high levels of anandamide are bad. Remember, there is high and there is too high, especially when combined with increased numbers of CB1 receptors in fatty tissue. It seems that we were created to take advantage of slightly elevated anandamide levels when in the growth phase of early childhood. However, when adding too much additional anandamide, one may cause a disbalance in the ECS leading to obesity later in life.

Obese individuals display an increased CB tone due to chronic activation of CB1 receptors. While initially it was believed that the endocannabinoid signaling system would only facilitate energy intake, scientists now know that the functions of endocannabinoids and CB1 receptors enhance energy storage into the adipose tissue and reduce energy expenditure by influencing both lipid and glucose metabolism.[423]

When mankind was created thousands of years ago, there was no processed food. People at that time had to work (burning many calories) to get their food which consisted mostly of plants and occasionally meat. This lifestyle supported the ECS, and in turn, the ECS supported that lifestyle. The reason that the ECS includes endocannabinoids such as anandamide, who to a certain extent preserve fat, was likely to support the body in times of famine.

But today's lack of movement combined with overindulgence of unhealthy, sugar-rich nutrition likely overloads these safeguards intended to increase survival in ancient times. As result, we lost some of the balancing effects of the ECS. We should not just consume CBD thinking it is a quick fix for a bad lifestyle. I call upon every one of you to start exercising and eating healthier. Then CBD will be able to support homeostasis rather than just cover up some symptoms.

I mentioned earlier that the precursor of anandamide and 2-AG is arachidonic acid (AA). AA, an omega-6 polyunsaturated fatty acid, can be metabolized into inflammatory compounds such as prostaglandins and leukotrienes as well as anti-inflammatory compounds. I also mentioned that hemp seeds have an optimal ratio of omega-6 to omega-3 and are hence very healthy.

Omega-3 fatty acids EPA (eicosapentaenoic acid) and DHA (docosahexaenoic acid) respectively reduce the amount of AA in the body and hence indirectly increase CB receptor functionality. They also seem to increase the amount of CB1 and CB2 receptors. And even metabolites of EPA and DHA have shown to have a high affinity for CB1 receptors. This is yet another indication that healthy food collaborates with our ECS.

It is also interesting to know that there is a difference between white adipose tissue (white fat cells) and brown adipose tissue. While white fat cells serve mostly as storage for energy in the form of calories, brown fat cells are used to burn fat and create heat in the process. [424] While white adipose tissue (WAT) and brown adipose tissue (BAT) are both involved in energy balance, they are characterized by different anatomical locations, morphological structures, functions, and regulations.

Recently, brown-like adipocytes were discovered in WAT. These brown-like adipocytes that appear in WAT are called beige or brite adipocytes. Interestingly, these beige/brite cells resemble white fat cells in the basal state, but they respond to cold stimuli with increased levels of thermogenic genes and increased respiration rates. The response of such types of WAT to thermogenic stimuli is called "browning."

The current epidemic of obesity has increased the interest in studying fat formation (adipogenesis), especially in beige/brite cells.[425] BATs are known to use glucose and triglycerides from the blood to increase the temperature in the body. So, the potential of BAT activity in protection against obesity and metabolic syndrome has been recognized.[426] Acute and repeated mild cold exposures of 17-19°C in adult humans increase BAT volume and activity. This is a natural method for increasing energy expenditure, i.e. supporting weight loss.[427]

So, what does all this WAT and BAT talk have to do with the endocannabinoid system? Research has shown that cold temperatures increase the endocannabinoid tone.[428] One study demonstrated the increase in density of CB1 receptors in the amygdala, a part of the brain located close to the hippocampus. Both the hippocampus and amygdala are involved in memory and emotions. It is interesting to note that metabolism, fat burning, and fat storage are connected to emotions and memory via up- or down-regulation of CB1 receptors especially in this part of the brain.

And now comes the very interesting part since CBD only very weakly influences these CB1 receptors in the brain, if at all. CBD itself has shown to be involved in browning of white adipocytes, augmentation of lipolysis (breakdown of fatty tissue), thermogenesis (maintenance of proper body temperatures), and reduction of lipogenesis (formation of fatty tissue). [429] And browning of fat is an efficient way to increase whole brown fat activity, which increases the burning of calories from fat.[430]

In other words, CBD by itself could be a potentially promising natural therapeutic agent for the prevention or treatment of obesity. In light of the ongoing obesity epidemic, these findings are of utmost importance and add an entirely new angle in regard to the benefits of CBD consumption. Who would have thought that adding CBD to your daily supplementation regimen could help you with weight loss or with maintaining your optimal body weight? The implications of this are far reaching.

Take Away Message
- Pharmacokinetics describes the ways in which drugs move through the body.
- Humans and animals can absorb CBD in a variety of ways involving different organ systems. Most common forms of intake of CBD are oral, sublingual/intra-oral, and topical/transdermal.
- Oral application and swallowing of CBD have a very low bioavailability.
- The absorption through the gut wall can be increased when combining CBD with other substances such as olive oil, sesame oil, or turmeric.
- The human brain contains an estimated 100 billion neural cells and around 85 billion glia-type cells.
- Neurons express mostly CB1 cannabinoid receptors, while glial cells express CB2
- The brain protects itself from being invaded by toxins present in the blood by creating and maintaining the

blood-brain-barrier. CBD preserves the functionality of the blood-brain-barrier.

- The endocannabinoid system plays a critical role in the regulation of emotions.
- The microbiome has also been called "the last undiscovered human organ".
- Cannabinoids inhibit gastric and intestinal motility through activation of enteric CB1 receptors
- Gut motility is one of the ways that the brain can control and influence bacterial composition in the gut.
- The ECS is involved in numerous biological processes including control of gut inflammation and gut-barrier function.
- Your lifestyle, food intake, physical activity, gut, microbiome, brain, and ECS are completely connected and any disturbance will have health consequences.
- CBD has a relaxing effect.
- A hyperactive ECS contributes to visceral fat accumulation and obesity.
- Acute aerobic exercise activates the ECS in physically active individuals.
- Athletes could benefit from CBD because it supports elevated levels of anandamide.
- About a third of today's world population is currently obese.
- Our endocannabinoid system was identified to include a group of molecules that significantly contributes to metabolic control and therefore weight control.
- CBD itself has shown to be involved in increasing the burning of calories from fat.
- CBD by itself could be a potentially promising natural therapeutic agent for the prevention or treatment of obesity.

Current Medical Research on CBD

Many patients suffering from pathological conditions start turning towards CBD. They recognized that medical drugs might help, however that help comes with a price tag, and not just in dollars. Often, the intake of a drug results in some side effects which then in turn must be treated by prescribing even more drugs. This is one of the hallmarks of so-called modern medicine. Not often enough do healthcare providers search for the cause of a pathological condition. Diagnosis is key and the next step is immediate treatment.

Wouldn't it be better to find and eliminate the root cause? That would remove the need for medical drugs in the first place. Many patients realized that they are caught in a vicious cycle and are looking for alternatives, and CBD could be one. In fact, almost 62% of CBD users reported using CBD to treat a medical condition.[431]

The top three medical conditions treated were pain, anxiety, and depression. The same authors found that 36% of respondents reported that CBD treats their medical condition(s) "very well by itself," while only 4.30% reported "not very well." Over 74% of respondents reported using CBD daily or more than daily.

Because of its safety profile and the many benefits CBD offers, patients seem to prefer CBD to traditional medications. According to one study, CBD is being used to replace traditional medicines, with 42% of respondents stopping their use of other medications to treat conditions including anxiety, insomnia, joint pain and inflammation, as well as depression. Respondents overwhelmingly preferred CBD derived from terpene-rich marijuana to CBD derived from industrial hemp. Only 9% of respondents indicated using hemp-derived CBD exclusively.[432]

In 2018, the FDA approved CBD for the treatment of two rare pediatric seizure disorders. As of the writing of this book, no other medical application for CBD has yet been approved. CBD is still classified by the FDA as a drug and has not yet received the official status of a dietary supplement. The FDA is still in the process of figuring out how to deal with CBD consumption and more important, how to regulate it.

Let's summarize some of the studies evaluating CBD consumption for medical conditions. This chapter, and the book, is in no way intended to give you medical recommendations. Please always contact your physician and healthcare provider when considering use of any natural products against any disease.

Always consider the potential interaction of natural products with any medications you might take. And while many studies are ongoing, and basically all results paint a very positive picture of use of CBD for various diseases, we all have to realize that to date, CBD, like many other natural products, is not approved to diagnose, prevent, treat, or cure any disease. And because CBD was banned for basically 100 years and only recently became available to the public, medical literature lacks results from long-term intake of CBD products.

CBD and Neurological Problems

Memory, mood stability, cognitive function, sleep, and many brain processes are vital for a happy life. According to the World Health Organization, mental health disorders are one of the leading causes of disability worldwide.[433] The WHO also stated recently that the burden of mental disorders continues to grow, with significant impacts on health, major social and human rights, and economies in all countries of the world.[434]

It is well known by now that CBD has neuroprotective and anti-inflammatory effects. As just mentioned, in 2018, the FDA approved CBD as a medical drug against two rare and severe forms of pediatric seizures called Lennox-Gastaut syndrome and Dravet syndrome.[435] Initial results of the studies investigating such patients revealed that CBD reduced seizure frequency and had an adequate safety profile in children and young adults with highly treatment-resistant epilepsy.[436] Several studies to treat other forms of seizures such as refractory epileptic encephalopathy are currently on the way.[437]

The exact antiepileptic mechanisms of CBD are not yet known. However, researchers suspect that the orphan G-protein-coupled receptor GPR55, the transient receptor potential of vanilloid type-1 channels TRPV, the 5-HT1a receptor, and the α3 and α1 glycine receptors are involved.[438] As you can see, trying to explain how CBD works via receptors is a little more complicated than just assuming it works by influencing either CB1 or CB2 receptors.

A variety of mechanisms have been suggested to be at play in regard to CBD and neurological disorders. Acute anxiolytic (anxiety reducing) and antidepressant-like effects seem to rely mainly on the interaction with serotonin 5-HT1A receptors in the brain. Other benefits such as anti-compulsive effects, increased extinction of bad memories, and facilitation of adult neurogenesis could depend on increased anandamide levels.

Finally, activation of TRPV1 channels are likely the reason for the antipsychotic effect observed with CBD.[439] But other mechanisms such as inhibiting the uptake of the neurotransmitter adenosine, binding to CB1, CB2, GRP55, and PPARγ receptors could also be behind the beneficial effects of CBD in neurological diseases.

CBD exerts positive pharmacological effects in ischemic stroke and other chronic diseases, including Parkinson's disease, Alzheimer's disease, and rheumatoid arthritis.[440] The same authors also mentioned that the brain-protective action of CBD is CB1 receptor-independent and long-lasting. Studies have also confirmed that CBD can be a safe and well-tolerated alternative treatment for schizophrenia.[441,442]

One review described the ability of CBD to reduce reactive gliosis (inflammation of certain brain cells responsible for cleaning the brain and creating new brain pathways) and the neuroinflammatory response, as well as to promote neurogenesis (the new formation of brain tissue and brain pathways). Importantly, CBD also reversed and prevented the development of cognitive deficits in Alzheimer's models.[443]

In clinical trials, CBD has shown the ability to reverse and even prevent the development of Alzheimer's negative impact.[444] A review of this topic in 2012 found that CBD promotes the growth and development of brain cells, which were shown to reduce the decline of memory and other brain functions.[445] The same authors just recently found that CBD possesses neuroprotective, antioxidant, and anti-inflammatory properties and reduces amyloid-β production and tau hyperphosphorylation, two important processes in Alzheimer's.[446]

In fact, one of the hallmarks of Alzheimer's disease is the accumulation of amyloid plaques between nerve cells in the brain. This highlights that CBD not only works through supporting and protecting brain nerves but also through keeping the brain clean of amyloids.

In summary, CBD supports healthy brain function through a combination of anxiolytic, anti-psychotic, and neuroprotective effects. CBD also influences the microbiome in a positive way and decreases inflammation in the gut. Why would that be important? Because there is a very close connection between gut health, the microbiome, and brain health. CBD can influence the brain and the gut, displaying its importance for homeostasis of both.

CBD and Sleep

Lack of sleep has dire consequences on overall health and quality-of-life.[447] Problems with falling asleep or daytime sleepiness affect approximately 35- 40% of the U.S. adult population annually and are a significant cause of morbidity (sickness) and mortality (death.[448] In addition, sleep problems are likely to rise due to the rapid advent of a 24/7 society involving round-the-clock activities and increased nighttime use of TV, internet, and mobile phones.[449] Sleep disorders are so common that the International Classification of Sleep Disorders now distinguishes more than 80 different ones.

The hypnogenic/sleep-promoting properties of marijuana have been recognized for centuries.[450] A study involving 72 adults presenting with anxiety or poor sleep found that anxiety scores decreased within the first month in 79.2% of the patients receiving CBD and remained decreased during the study duration. Sleep scores improved within the first month in 66.7% of the patients but fluctuated over time.[451]

It was suggested that CBD plays a role in the treatment of sleep disorders because it can improve certain phases like Rapid Eye Movement (REM) sleep and reduce excessive daytime sleepiness.[452] Adults spend about 20-30% of their sleep in REM, while babies can spend up to 50% in this stage.

Other studies showed that systemic acute administration of CBD appears to increase total sleep time.[453] One case report described how CBD oil was used as a safe treatment for reducing anxiety and improving sleep in a young girl with posttraumatic stress disorder.[454]

While many studies found positive effects of CBD in regard to supporting sleep, it should also be mentioned that one particular study looked at the effect of CBD on sleep-wake cycles in volunteers and found no difference between the groups receiving CBD or a placebo.[455] The caveat here is that healthy volunteers were used and not people with sleep disturbances. Perhaps CBD works for those with sleep disorders while not negatively affecting healthy people. This could be an important finding for those who use CBD for other reasons than supporting sleep.

The fact that CBD might actually increase alertness was mostly supported by animal studies.[456] In humans, one study on insomniac volunteers receiving 160mg CBD reported that these patients slept significantly more than those receiving placebo.[457] In addition, the volunteers also reported significantly less dream recall which indicates deeper sleep cycles.

While there is still discussion on whether CBD increases alertness and could be used to counteract daytime sleepiness or whether it increases sleep and deepens sleep quality,[458] it is my personal experience that CBD blended with essential oils can be very powerful in supporting healthy sleep. This entire discussion again highlights the duality of the effects of CBD. It is once more the concept of homeostasis, in this case to optimize sleep-wake balance, depending on what is needed.

CBD and Anxiety

Up to 34% of the population suffers from anxiety disorders, including panic disorders with or without agoraphobia (fear of places and situations that might cause panic, helplessness, or embarrassment), generalized anxiety disorders, social anxiety disorders, specific phobias, and separation anxiety disorders.[459]

These conditions are associated with immense health care costs and a high burden of disease, severely lowering quality-of-life for those affected. Anxiety disorders also lead to the onset, persistence, or severity of secondary disorders such as mood and substance abuse disorders.[460]

Several reviews have confirmed the beneficial effects of CBD on anxiety. [461,462,463] Acute administration of CBD was beneficial for generalized anxiety, panic, social anxiety, obsessive-compulsive, and post-traumatic stress disorders.[464] CBD has shown to reduce anxiety and depression via activation of serotonergic 5-HT1A and other cannabinoid receptors when brains assess an initial response to threat. [465,466]

CBD also works on fear memory processing indicating that it reduces learned fear relevant to phobias and post-traumatic stress disorder. It does so by acutely reducing fear and fear memory while at the same time enhancing fear extinction, all important for lasting reduction of fear.[467,468,469] The use of CBD represents an interesting new natural way to approach such disorders.

Fear of public speaking is one of the most common anxieties and panic disorders. It affects many of us. Researchers demonstrated that a single oral dose of CBD (300mg) decreased anxiety from public speaking in healthy volunteers.[470] Another study with 24 volunteers revealed that oral pretreatment with 600mg CBD significantly reduced anxiety, cognitive impairment, and discomfort in speech performance, and significantly decreased negative alert reactions to the upcoming speech.[471] Anxiety is among the top reasons for CBD use.

CBD and Pain

Over 50% of today's doctor visits are related to joint or back pain.[472] In the U.S. for example, at least 25% of patients suffer from back pain.[473] Lower back pain alone was ranked to be fifth in the reasons to make a doctor's appointment and therefore represents a major reason for all physician office visits.[474] In the U.S., it has been reported that 126.1 million adults experienced some pain in the previous three months. About 25 million adults (11.2%) are suffering from daily chronic pain and 23.4 million (10.3%) reported a lot of pain overall.[475]

The best-known painkiller among the cannabinoids is THC supported by CBD.[476] It has been suggested that CBD may enhance THC's analgesic effects by primarily prolonging THC's duration of action.[477] CB1 and other types of receptors in the brain, spinal cord, and peripheral nervous system interact with the cannabinoids in order to control pain.[478]

A group of researchers found that CBD can act via TRPV1 receptors, as mentioned earlier, and thereby alleviating antihyperalgesic action (counteract an exacerbated response to pain).[479] Natural phytocannabinoids and synthetic derivatives have produced clear activity in a variety of pain conditions. These effects are the result of both inhibition of pain pathway signaling (mostly CB1) and anti-inflammatory effects (mostly CB2).[480]

In addition, CB2 receptors also contribute to pain reduction by inhibiting the release of proinflammatory factors near pain perceiving neuron endings.[481] Basically, the activation of CB2 receptors can either directly decrease pain perception or indirectly diminish pain by decreasing pain-related inflammatory compounds close to the nerves responsible for pain perception.

Another study found that cannabinoids suppress inflammatory and neuropathic pain by targeting α3 glycine receptors.[482] As you can see, the ECS is complicated and many receptor types such as CB1 and CB2, TRPV, GRP55, α3 glycine, as well as probably other cannabinoid receptors are involved in reducing pain and inflammation.

Marijuana-based medicines have also shown to increase the number of people achieving 50% or greater pain relief compared with a placebo.[483] Transdermal/topical CBD gel significantly reduced joint swelling, limb posture scores as a rating of spontaneous pain, immune cell infiltration, and thickening of the synovial membrane in a dose-dependent manner, making it an interesting topical treatment modality for pain without having any evident side effects.[484]

One study looked at the effects of CBD and/or THC in patients with neurogenic symptoms from multiple sclerosis, spinal cord injury, and limb amputation unresponsive to standard treatment. The results showed that both CBD and THC were significantly superior in treating pain compared to placebo.[485] In addition, symptoms such as impaired bladder control, muscle spasms and spasticity, often seen in this patient population, were also improved.

Another study reported that topical transdermal delivery of CBD decreased alcohol-related neurodegeneration and therefore potentially prevents or decreases pain in such conditions.[486] Yet another study found that topical CBD application resulted in relief of arthritis pain-related behaviors and inflammation without evident side-effects.[487] CBD, through its combined immunosuppressive and anti-inflammatory actions, has a potent anti-arthritic effect.[488] CBD administration was also able to decrease chemotherapy-induced neuropathic pain in cancer patients while not decreasing the activity of the chemotherapy.[489]

There is plenty of evidence that CBD and other cannabinoids are able to reduce painful conditions. It has also been my personal experience that topical and sublingual administrations of CBD with and without essential oils were able to support a life free of or with significantly reduced pain.

CBD and Skin

The skin is the body's largest organ. The skin primarily establishes, controls, and transmits contacts with the external world. In addition, the skin acts as a barrier and protects our body from deleterious environmental impacts (physical, chemical, and microbiological) and is well-known as being crucial for the maintenance of temperature, electrolyte and fluid balance, as well as immune functions.[490]

Current research shows that the skin also operates as a huge and highly active biofactory for the synthesis, processing, and/or metabolism of an astounding range of structural proteins, lipids, and other compounds. It is now becoming appreciated that the skin is an integral component of the immune, nervous, and endocrine systems. The skin also plays a huge role in beauty,[491] antiaging,[492] and one's perception of health of another person.[493]

We now know that the ECS is also found in the skin. Its role there is likely to control biological processes such as proliferation, growth, differentiation, and apoptosis/death of skin cells. It may also balance inflammatory cytokines and hormone production of various cell types of the skin and appendages, such as the hair follicle and sebaceous glands. It seems that the main physiological function of the skin-based ECS is to control the proper and well-balanced creation, survival, and immune function of skin cells.[494]

Newer findings point towards the involvement of the skin in neuro-immuno-endocrine organ function. The interactive network between cutaneous nerves, the neuroendocrine axis, and the immune system has been well established.[495] The interaction between nerves in the skin and cell growth, immunity, inflammation, pruritus, and wound healing is a new field of exploration. So is the science of how the microbiome can influence the skin and vice versa.

Research showed that a dense network of sensory nerves is capable of releasing over 50 neuropeptides (small proteins with function in the nervous system), thereby modulating inflammation, cell growth, and the immune responses in the skin.[496] The ECS of the skin has shown to do the same. Is there a connection?

It was even postulated that cutaneous cannabinoids, also named "c[ut]annabinoids," are deeply involved in the maintenance of skin homeostasis, barrier formation, and regeneration.[497] Neuropeptides are synthesized locally in skin cells and are transported by nerve fibers or immune cells to their targets.

Several neuropeptides cause an inflammatory response with edema and erythema (reddening of the skin), induce the release of histamine by mastocytes (a reaction that makes you itch and swell locally), regulate cutaneous blood flow, participate in sweat regulation, and induce pain.[498] They also exert their action over several cells that participate in immunity, thereby inhibiting or stimulating inflammatory mechanisms.

Some receptors for neuropeptides were found on epidermal skin cells. The epidermis is the outer layer of the skin. Studies indicate that these neuropeptides are involved in inducing or improving skin lesions like psoriasis, atopic eczema, alopecia areata (loss of hair), vitiligo (skin condition with loss of pigmentation), pruritus (itching), hypertrophic scars, and other conditions.

So how do these neuropeptides and the skin know how to act? It is again the duality of body systems. New research is now concentrating on understanding the possible connections between the skin and the ECS, as well as how the ECS supports homeostasis of the skin and the closely related immune system.

Some of the skin nerves are olfactory nerves (smell nerves).[499] Yes, your skin as well as other organs can in fact smell odors and use the language of scents to, for example, support wound healing. In addition, taste receptors have also been found in the skin and seem to also be involved in wound healing. [500]

The functional implications of these taste receptors being widely dispersed in various organs including the skin shed a new light on several concepts used in ayurvedic pharmacology (dravyaguna vijnana), such as taste (rasa), post-digestive effect (vipaka), qualities (guna), and energetic nature (virya).[501] To make it more interesting, CB2 receptors have also been found to be upregulated during wound healing.[502]

Isn't that fascinating? This is where I, as a traditionally trained physician, had to make huge changes in my thinking. The connections between homeostasis, natural products, scents from essential oils, the microbiome, and all organ systems suddenly became clear. This is the reason why I stepped back and now try to see everything from a holistic viewpoint instead of from a highly specialized and narrow view.

At higher doses, CBD was found to inhibit the synthesis of lipids in sebocytes (any of the cells that make up the sebaceous glands and secrete sebum) and to produce apoptosis (suicide of some of the overactive sebum gland cells) in acne.[503] CBD, in addition to its anti-inflammatory and bacteriostatic effects, is a TRPV4 agonist that works as a highly effective sebum reducing agent in acne.[504]

Results of another study showed that cannabinoids inhibit keratinocytes (cells that produce hard skin layers), and therefore support a potential role for cannabinoids in the treatment of psoriasis.[505,506] Moreover, based on their remarkable anti-inflammatory actions, phytocannabinoids could be efficient, yet safe innovative tools in the management of cutaneous inflammations.[507]

Anandamide and 2-AG have also been found in hair follicles. In fact, full-spectrum hemp oil containing cannabinoids such as CBD and THC are marketed as an effective cosmetic treatment for hair, with claims that direct application of the oil to hair has moisturizing benefits, can aid hair growth, may protect the hair and aid in damage repair, and add shine to the hair.[508] It has been shown that the ECS and endocannabinoids have been implemented in regulating hair follicle activity.[509]

However, a group of scientists found that activation of CB1 receptors in hair follicles inhibited hair growth.[510] These findings were confirmed by another study looking at the effects of cannabinoids on transient potential vanilloid 1 and 3 (TRPV1 and TRPV3) receptors.[511,512] And while the anti-inflammatory effects of CBD could support hair growth, it is not yet clear how this would counteract CB1 receptor activation with inhibition of hair growth. One thing is clear however, the ECS is involved.

It is also noteworthy that the abuse of synthetic, hyper-potent cannabinoids such as Bonsai, fake weed, K2, and Jamaica can result in dermatological disorders, such as premature skin aging, hair loss and graying, or acne.[513] This is likely caused by the blockage or over-activation of endocannabinoid receptors in the skin and hair by these dangerous synthetic drugs.

Our endocannabinoid anandamide is also involved in the activation of our color pigment-producing cells called melanocytes.[514] Interestingly, another connection between black pigment and our ECS is demonstrated by the fact that black truffles can produce anandamide. This could explain why certain people like to eat them. It has been suggested that they, and the animals used to find these truffles, get a high from the anandamide consumed.[515]

Anandamide and the activation of cannabinoid receptors in the skin, especially receptors of the transient receptor potential (TRP) family, are part of the sensation you feel on your skin.[516] This shows how the ECS helps our body to connect to stimuli from outside the body to help us achieve homeostasis, not just in our body alone but probably also with our environment.

Preliminary studies in Europe showed that after the first seven days of topical treatment with CBD-based lotion, 85.71% of the women reported an improvement of their skin. At the end of the 14 days of treatment, 100% of the women said they noticed an improvement. The trial also found that 81% of the participants specifically noticed an improvement in skin texture as well as an improvement in the appearance of fine lines and wrinkles around the mouth.[517] However, it is not clear what other ingredients besides CBD were mixed into the lotion.

In summary, the important role of the ECS in the skin has been well established. Cannabinoid signaling is a key contributor to cutaneous homeostasis. CBD and other cannabinoids are novel tools to support healthy skin and antiaging.

CBD and Cancer

In the U.S., cardiovascular diseases are still the leading cause of death, with cancer second. In some states, cancer is now number one.[518] Worldwide, cancer is still second after cardiovascular diseases. A study involving over 500 researchers representing over 300 institutions and 50 countries revealed that cancer mortality decreased between 2005 and 2015 despite the global incidence rates of cancer increasing during this period.[519]

So, fewer people are dying from cancer but more are getting it. The most common cancers are prostate, lung, and colorectal cancer in males, and breast, colorectal, and lung cancer in females. When it comes to mortality, leading causes of cancer deaths are lung, liver, and gastric cancer in males and breast, lung, and colorectal cancer in females.[520]

Emerging evidence suggests that compounds able to bind to cannabinoid receptors expressed by tumor cells offer a novel strategy to treat cancer. Several preclinical studies propose that cannabinoids, synthetic cannabinoids, and endocannabinoids have anti-cancer effects in vitro studies (in cell lines) against lung carcinoma, gliomas, thyroid epithelioma, lymphoma, skin carcinoma, uterine carcinoma, breast cancer, prostate carcinoma, pancreatic cancer and neuroblastoma.[521]

In vivo studies (in animals) are confirming these findings. In addition, cannabinoids are also used in cancer medicine to treat nausea and vomiting associated with chemo- or radiotherapy, and for appetite stimulation, pain relief, mood elevation, and insomnia in cancer patients.[522]

It seems that our own body created a system by which it can attack cancer cells and even prevent them from migrating and causing metastasis (development of secondary malignant growths at a distance from a primary site of cancer).[523] The endocannabinoid system is like having built-in chemotherapy without deleterious effects on the immune system.

In fact, the immune system is supported while cancer cells are attacked. Both CB1 and CB2 receptors are involved in the fight against cancer. However, it seems that CB1 and possibly other receptors play a larger role.

Upregulated expression of CB receptors and elevated endocannabinoid levels have been found in a variety of cancer cells such as skin, prostate, and colon cancer, hepatocellular carcinoma, endometrial sarcoma, glioblastoma multiforme, meningioma and pituitary adenoma, Hodgkin's lymphoma, as well as chemically induced liver carcinoma and mantel cell lymphoma.[524]

One study showed that anandamide blocks human breast cancer cell proliferation through CB1-like receptor-mediated cancer inhibition.[525] Human melanomas also express CB1 and CB2 receptors and activation of these receptors decreased growth, proliferation, angiogenesis (the growth of new blood vessels into a cancer), and metastasis while increasing apoptosis.[526]

Many studies in the past looked only at the effects of marijuana on cancer. THC and other cannabinoids found in marijuana are long known for their anticancer properties as shown in breast,[527] prostate,[528] lung, skin, and many other types of cancers.[529] Cannabinoids have also been used in combination with chemotherapy to fight pancreatic cancer, for example.[530]

But evidence that CBD is an important tool in fighting cancers, whether through activation of CB receptors in cancer cells or by producing elevated levels of endocannabinoids such as anandamide with anticancer activity, is mounting. A group of authors demonstrated that CBD was able to produce a significant antitumor activity both in vitro and in vivo, thus suggesting it as an antineoplastic (anti-cancer) agent.[531]

It was also mentioned earlier in this book that CBD can activate peroxisome proliferator-activated receptor -γ (PPARγ) receptors. PPARγ stimulation may kill cancer cells without toxicity to normal cells.[532] PPARγ has been identified in many cancers including those affecting the brain, and its activation inhibits tumor cell growth.

CBD has also been shown to inhibit growth of lung cancer cells by influencing COX-2 and PPAR-γ receptors.[533] Other studies revealed that blocking the enzyme FAAH increases the levels of anandamide which ultimately leads to cell cycle arrest and death of the cancer cells. [534,535]

Let's translate that. We know that CBD elevates anandamide because it inhibits FAAH, the breakdown enzyme of that endocannabinoid. Anandamide has shown to influence cancer cells by inhibiting important growth factor receptors on their surface. This leads to a halt in growth and the suicide of cancer cells. The current literature on CBD and other cannabinoids and cancer is vast.

Several studies also confirmed the palliative value CBD and other cannabinoids have for cancer patients.[536,537,538] Palliative care means treating only the symptoms, like pain or nausea, without affecting the cancer directly. One study found that cannabinoids are safe in cancer patients with pain not completely relieved by opioids when used in moderate doses.[539]

Another study revealed that cannabinoids were more effective compared to other anti-nausea medications, and also the number of doses could be reduced in patients with chemotherapy-induced nausea and vomiting.[540] It was also interesting that patients in this study preferred cannabinoids over traditional anti-nausea drugs for future rounds of chemotherapy. This could be related to the mood enhancing effects of cannabinoids which are not seen in normal anti-nausea drugs.

In summary, cannabinoids have an increasing role in the treatment and palliative care of cancer patients. The medical literature is vast and growing fast when it comes to cannabinoids and cancer. We need to be careful not to automatically conclude that CBD alone is always the miraculous compound. Now that CBD has been de-scheduled, it will be easier to conduct studies with CBD alone, and it will be very interesting to see what future CBD studies in cancer care will show. The evidence we have right now certainly points towards positive effects of CBD in cancer patients, in the treatment of both the cancer itself as well as the symptoms of the disease.

CBD and Autoimmune Diseases

Autoimmune diseases are among the leading causes of death among young and middle-aged women in the United States. It was previously estimated that about 500 per 100,000 people suffer from these conditions.[541] However, newer data suggest that up to 10% of the population have them.[542]

Examples of the more than two dozen autoimmune diseases include Grave's disease, rheumatoid arthritis, Hashimoto thyroiditis, rheumatoid arthritis, Type I diabetes, Sjogren syndrome, primary systemic vasculitis, systemic sclerosis, systemic lupus erythematosus, psoriasis, myasthenia gravis, primary biliary cirrhosis, Crohn's disease, ulcerative colitis, Goodpasture's syndrome, idiopathic thrombocytopenia purpura, relapsing polychondritis, Guillain-Barre syndrome, Miller-Fisher syndrome, and multiple sclerosis.

It is estimated that over one million new cases of these autoimmune diseases occur in the United States every five years. Women are at a 2.7 times greater risk than men to acquire an autoimmune disease.[543] Scientists and clinicians observed a dramatic increase of allergic and autoimmune diseases in past decades.[544]

Autoimmune problems are known to occur with increased frequency in patients that already suffer from at least one other autoimmune disease, indicating a dysregulation in homeostasis.[545] Both genetics and epigenetics, the influence of the environment and lifestyle on genes, contribute to the occurrence of autoimmune diseases.[546] The environment can contribute to autoimmunity by modifying gene expression through epigenetic mechanisms. One more reason to avoid the chemicals and toxins negatively influencing our daily life.

Cannabinoids have shown to be effective in reducing inflammation in arthritis and multiple sclerosis, and to have a positive effect on neuropathic pain and on Type I diabetes mellitus. They are effective as treatment for fibromyalgia and have shown to have an anti-fibrotic effect in scleroderma.[547] These findings highlight the importance of the ECS in regulating an immune system that went into overdrive.

As mentioned earlier, CB2 receptors are known to be mostly found in the immune system.[548] Activation of CB2 receptors results in a reduction of inflammation but also in a calming of an immune system in overdrive. These receptors are an important part of regulating and balancing immune responses. Sometimes, this has to be done through immune suppression.

CB2 receptor activation has a protective effect during chronic autoimmune-induced liver diseases.[549] Scientists found that elevated anandamide levels, such as seen after CBD administration, reduce autoimmune hepatitis by suppressing inflammatory cytokine levels.[550] Another study revealed the importance of CB2 receptors in the prevention or treatment of multiple sclerosis.[551]

Multiple sclerosis is characterized by autoimmune damage to nerve tissue through demyelination of nerve fibers and axons in the brain and nerves. It means that antibodies produced by the body attack one's own nerve sheaths, kind of a collateral damage by friendly fire. This results in symptoms like muscle spasms, tremor, ataxia (inability to walk), weakness or paralysis, constipation, and loss of bladder control.[552] Early studies in the 90s demonstrated that marijuana use improved symptoms such as spasticity, pain, tremors, and depression in more than 90% of patients.[553]

Newer studies found that CBD could decrease the number and migration of inflammatory cells, lowering the inflammatory damage seen in multiple sclerosis.[554,555,556] The significance of CBD in regulating immune response is also shown by its importance in regulating inflammatory compounds within the body.[557]

CBD has also shown to lower autoimmune diabetic disorders by supporting immunomodulatory mechanisms.[558] Several clinical trials for multiple sclerosis, inflammatory bowel disease, and fibromyalgia suggest marijuana' effectiveness as an immune-modulator.[559] CBD also works against autoimmune rheumatoid arthritis.[560] As little as 6.2mg of CBD per day resulted in an improvement of joint inflammation as seen in rheumatoid arthritis and similar conditions.[561]

CBD reduces intestinal inflammation in inflammatory bowel diseases.[562] It is also clear that the microbiome plays a central role in the autoimmunity of the gut.[563] For example, researchers found a close relationship between systemic lupus erythematosus and an alteration of the intestinal microbiome.[564] Again, the close connection between CBD, ECS, and the microbiome have been mentioned in several studies.[565]

This discussion about autoimmune conditions and CBD highlights once more the duality of action of cannabinoids. On one hand they have shown to support the immune system by strengthening it, and on the other hand they cause immune suppression in patients with autoimmune diseases in order to rebalance an immune system gone wild. It is all about homeostasis!

CBD and Osteopenia/Osteoporosis

Osteoporosis, the extreme form of osteopenia, is the most common bone disease in humans. With an aging population and longer life span, osteoporosis is increasingly becoming a global epidemic.[566] Currently, it has been estimated that more than 200 million women globally are suffering from osteoporosis. According to recent statistics from the International Osteoporosis Foundation, one in three women over the age of 50 worldwide, and one in five men, will experience osteoporotic fractures in their lifetime.[567]

Annually, osteoporosis causes more than 8.9 million fractures across the globe, resulting in an osteoporotic fracture every three seconds. Among those, forearm, hip, and back fractures are almost equally represented.[568] Once a person suffers one fracture, the risk of a subsequent fracture related to osteoporosis increases by 86%.[569] Osteoporotic fractures represent a significant cause of morbidity and mortality, particularly in developed countries. The prevention and treatment of osteoporosis is very important.

Luckily, CBD and the ECS are involved in the maintenance of bone mass. A study showed that activation of CB2 receptors in the bone is extremely important for healthy bone mass.[570] This study also revealed that activation of CB2 receptors enhances osteoblast number and activity while restraining osteoclasts.

Osteoblasts are cells in charge of building new bone, while osteoclasts break down bone. So the activation of CB2 receptors in the bone leads to more bone formation and less bone breakdown. These results demonstrate that the endocannabinoid system is essential for the maintenance of normal bone mass by osteoblastic and osteoclastic CB2 signaling.

Other authors confirmed the importance of CB2 receptors in the regulation of osteoblast and osteoclast formation, indicating that these receptors are a very interesting target for potential new drugs for bone loss prevention.[571] In fact, it could be shown that CB2 receptors are expressed (formed) directly in osteoblasts and osteoclasts, thereby stimulating bone formation while inhibiting bone resorption.[572]

An interesting study revealed that CBD leads to improvement in fracture healing.[573] The authors looked at the mechanism of fracture healing and found that CBD had a critical role in collagen crosslinking in the bone, improving the bone formation across the fracture. Another study showed that CBD administration attenuated sublesional bone loss after spinal cord injury.[574] Patients with spinal cord injury typically experience severe loss of bone mineral below the level of the spinal cord lesion. It seems that CBD could help prevent such bone loss.

Of equal importance is the fact that cannabinoids regulate tumor-bone cell interactions via CB2 receptors.[575] The authors of that study suggest that agents that target CB2 receptors in the skeleton have potential efficacy in the reduction of skeletal complications associated with cancer. In addition, cannabinoids support the body in its fight against cancer growth, bone loss (as seen in certain cancer metastasis into the bone), and pain from cancerous bone lesions.[576]

There is a reason that anandamide and 2-AG are present in the bone at levels nearly as high as the brain.[577] We know that our endocannabinoids anandamide and 2-AG, phytocannabinoids such as CBD, as well as CB1 and CB2 receptors in bone cells, play an important role in the homeostasis of healthy bone.

CBD and Cardiovascular Diseases

Cardiovascular diseases are still the leading cause of mortality worldwide.[578] Ischemic heart disease including heart attacks, stroke, hypertension, and congestive heart failure make up about 80% of all cardiovascular diseases.[579] It is very clear that poor lifestyle choices are at the cause of most cardiovascular problems, and that better nutrition, exercise, and smoking cessation, just to name a few, could largely prevent these conditions.[580,581,582]

The ECS is widely distributed throughout the cardiovascular system highlighting the importance CBD and anandamide can have for better heart and blood vessel function. For example, anandamide plays a role in the cardiovascular system by lowering heart rate and blood pressure,[583] improving the lipid profiles and coronary blood flow, and increasing overall cardiac function.[584]

We know cannabinoids such as CBD can either inhibit or enhance certain effects, depending on what the body needs for homeostasis. This principle is no different in the cardiovascular system. For example, when blood pressure is too low (hypotension) such as when a body is in shock, endocannabinoids released within the blood improve the associated hypotension through CB1 receptor activation.

On the other hand, in conditions associated with high blood pressure (hypertension), there is evidence for down-regulation of expression of CB1 receptors. As a result of CB1 receptor antagonism, we see a reduction in blood pressure in obese, hypertensive, and diabetic patients.[585]

In the blood vessels, endocannabinoids cause vasorelaxation, the widening of blood vessels, through activation of multiple target sites, inhibition of calcium channels, activation of potassium channels, nitric oxide production, and the release of vasoactive substances. This results in the widening of the coronary arteries, important blood vessels of the heart, with consequent better oxygenation of the heart tissue.[586]

Overall, endocannabinoids such as anandamide have positive effects on CB2 receptors and negative effects on CB1 receptors, resulting in a decrease of progression of atherosclerosis (the calcification and stiffening of blood vessels).[587] It can therefore be concluded that CBD and the elevated anandamide levels produced by CBD have cardioprotective effects.[588]

CBD and Eye Diseases

Globally, there are an estimated 60 million people with pressure-related optic neuropathy and an estimated 8.4 million people who are blind as the result of glaucoma. These numbers are set to increase to 80 million and 11.2 million by 2020, making glaucoma the second leading cause of blindness around the world.[589]

Glaucoma causes optic nerve damage through high pressure within the eye, a condition called high intra-ocular pressure. Studies revealed that there is a wide distribution of cannabinoid CB1 receptors in both the anterior eye and the retina of humans.[590] These findings suggest that cannabinoids influence several different physiological functions in the human eye including the intraocular pressure.

In fact, cannabinoids effectively lower the intraocular pressure and have neuroprotective effects. A study in the 1970s already mentioned the eye pressure-lowering benefit (up to 30% lower) of smoking marijuana.[591] We now know that also CBD, cannabigerol, and endogenous cannabinoids such as anandamide and 2-AG all lower intraocular pressure.[592]

You read a little earlier that CBD and endocannabinoids lower blood pressure, and therefore have cardiovascular benefits. It would be easy to conclude that this blood pressure-lowering effect is the reason for lower eye pressure as well. However, the intraocular pressure-reducing effect does not seem to be related to a systemic reduction of arterial blood pressure.[593]

More recent research concentrated on two mechanisms: activation of CB1 receptors within the eye resulting in lower fluid production and direct neuroprotective effects of cannabinoids at the level of the optic nerve.[594,595] The combination of dryness of the eye and widening of the eye blood vessels is also believed to be the cause of redness of the eyes (conjunctivitis) when consuming marijuana products.[596]

Phytocannabinoids such as CBD, THC, and others either directly affect CB receptors in the eye or increase levels of anandamide and 2-AG which then influence ocular CB receptors or protect the optic nerve. Either way, the effect is a lowering of intraocular pressure and a protection of the optic nerve, both so important for prevention and treatment of glaucoma.

CBD and Addictions

Three million U.S. citizens and 16 million citizens worldwide have had or currently suffer from opioid addiction, and more than 500,000 people in the United States are dependent on heroin.[597] The mortality from opioid overdosing is high.[598] Deaths attributable to opioids increased 292% between 2001 and 2016, resulting in approximately 1.68 million person-years of life lost in 2016 alone. A staggering 20% of deaths in the age group of 20 to 35 involved opioids.[599]

In 2015, 63.1% of all drug overdose deaths in the U.S. were related to opioids.[600] As mentioned earlier, on average, 130 Americans die every day from an opioid overdose.[601] Because of these horrifying numbers, opioid overdose was declared a national emergency in the United States in 2017.

Mortality in opioid addiction comes partly from the dense representation of opioid receptors in the brainstem, an area responsible for many important functions of the body such as breathing, blood pressure, heart rate, and others. Activation of these receptors can provoke a stopping in breathing or a collapse in cardiovascular function and subsequently lead to death.

CBD is thought to modulate various neuronal circuits involved in drug addiction. We know that CBD acts with low affinity on CB1 and CB2 receptors, stimulates the TRVP1 receptors, inhibits the breakdown of anandamide by inhibiting FAAH, binds to 5-HT1a serotoninergic receptors, and influences GABA receptors. In addition, CBD also modulates μ and δ opioid receptors.[602] All of these receptors are involved in one way or another in addiction.

CBD interferes with brain reward mechanisms responsible for the desire to consume opioids.[603] CBD was also demonstrated to attenuate heroin-seeking behavior.[604] One case report describes a 19-year-old woman with marijuana withdrawal syndrome treated with CBD for 10 days. Daily symptom assessments demonstrated the absence of significant withdrawal, anxiety, and neurological symptoms during the treatment.[605]

CBD may have antagonistic effects at the CB1 receptors in the brain, as it was able to reduce the memory-impairing effects of THC.[606] This finding led to the recommendation that marijuana smokers should select strains that contain some CBD. The same group of authors also found that a higher ratio of CBD in marijuana strains was associated with lower ratings of pleasantness for the drug, potentially deceasing the addictive behavior of marijuana smokers.[607]

Another study evaluated the usefulness of CBD in reducing tobacco smoking addiction. The results revealed a significant reduction (approximately 40%) in the number of cigarettes smoked in the CBD inhaler group compared to the placebo group during the week of treatment.[608]

The role of CBD in alcohol addiction is still somewhat unclear.[609] However, a very recent review revealed that CBD had a neuroprotective effect against adverse alcohol consequences. CBD also diminished alcohol-induced hepatotoxicity such as alcohol-induced steatosis (alcoholic fatty liver). In addition, CBD reduced alcohol seeking, alcohol self-administration, and withdrawal-induced convulsions.[610]

All in all, CBD is a very interesting natural compound when it comes to addictions. Since there are very few CB receptors in the brainstem, neither CBD nor THC can elicit fatal complications. This is why, so far, no fatalities, besides accidental death when under the influence, have been attributed to marijuana smoking. Also, opioid abuse significantly decreased in states where recreational and medical marijuana is permitted.[611] I hope our politicians take note of such statistics and finally approve CBD for legal consumption without major restrictions in all 50 states.

Take Away Message

- Many patients suffering from pathological conditions start turning towards CBD.
- The FDA is still in the process of figuring out how to deal with CBD consumption and more important, how to regulate it.
- Please always contact your physician and healthcare provider when considering use of any natural products against any disease.
- CBD supports healthy brain function through a combination of anxiolytic, anti-psychotic, and neuroprotective effects.
- It is my personal experience that CBD blended with essential oils can be very powerful in supporting healthy sleep.
- Several reviews have confirmed the beneficial effects of CBD on anxiety, and it is among the top reasons for CBD use.
- It has been shown that the ECS and endocannabinoids have been implemented in regulating hair follicle activity.
- The important role of the ECS in the skin has been well established. CBD and other cannabinoids are novel tools to support healthy skin and antiaging.
- Emerging evidence suggests that compounds able to bind to cannabinoid receptors expressed by tumor cells offer a novel strategy to treat cancer.
- Both CB1 and CB2 receptors are involved in the fight against cancer. Cannabinoids have an increasing role in the treatment and palliative care of cancer patients.
- Activation of CB2 receptors results in a reduction of inflammation but also in a calming of an immune system in overdrive.
- The activation of CB2 receptors in the bone leads to more bone formation and less bone breakdown.

- The ECS is widely distributed throughout the cardiovascular system highlighting the importance CBD and anandamide can have for better heart and blood vessel function.
- Cannabinoids effectively lower the intraocular pressure and have neuroprotective effects on eyes.
- CBD is a very interesting natural compound when it comes to addictions.

Side Effects of CBD

A review conducted with 2,200 CBD users showed that the top five most frequently reported adverse effects were dry mouth (11.1% of users), euphoria (6.4%), hunger (6.4%), red eyes (2.7%), and sedation/fatigue (1.8%).[612] Just under 28.5% of medical users reported an adverse effect when compared with 34.6% of general health and well-being users.

Keep in mind that medical users are more likely to use higher doses and multiple routes of administration compared to wellness users. Another study found that most commonly reported side effects were tiredness, diarrhea, and changes of appetite/weight.[613] One single case of liver damage was mentioned in the same review. The authors concluded that in comparison with other drugs, CBD has a better side effect profile.

Since CBD has only been used by a larger number of people for a few years, we are missing long-term data in this regard. Recently during a public hearing, the FDA cited an increase in liver damage case reports when using CBD as an argument to put stricter controls on CBD[614]. However, when searching current medical literature, these anecdotal case reports are nowhere to be found.

The only related study presented at that hearing involved one group of researchers who studied the liver toxicity of CBD on rats. They found that under certain conditions, like when combined with the pharmaceutical drug acetaminophen, known as Tylenol, CBD could damage the liver. We will have to wait to get better data on this since acetaminophen itself is known to cause severe liver damage and even death. In fact, almost every study looking at CBD and the liver mentions its beneficial effects on this organ.

I previously discussed the interaction of CBD with the cytochrome enzyme system (CYP enzymes, especially CYP3A4) in the liver. By utilizing these enzymes and also by inhibiting some of them, CBD can interfere with the breakdown of other compounds such as prescription medications.[615,616]

Approximately 60% of clinically prescribed drugs are metabolized via CYP3A4. Significant drug-drug interactions have for example been reported when CBD is taken together with commonly prescribed psychotropic agents.[617] It is not always CBD that interacts with other drugs. Various drugs such as ketoconazol, itraconazol, ritonavir, and clarithromycin inhibit CYP3A4 in the liver and slow down the breakdown of CBD, increasing its amount in the blood.

In contrast, phenobarbital, rifampicin, carbamazepine, and phenytoin induce CYP3A4, causing reduced CBD bioavailability.[618] Specifically, Ketoconazol, an antifungal drug, almost doubles the blood content levels of CBD while rifampicin, an antibiotic, significantly reduced the amount of CBD in the blood.

One investigation with 10 patients using barbiturates found that CBD increased the bioavailability and elimination half-time of these drugs.[619] Barbiturates are used as anxiolytics, hypnotics, and anticonvulsants.

Therefore, there is an increased risk for over-sedation when combining CBD with this type of drug.

Another important interaction is that CBD inhibits the hepatic enzyme CYP2C9, reducing the metabolization of warfarin and diclofenac.[620] Warfarin is a very common blood thinner, and CBD consumption can increase the blood level of this medication, which increases the risk of bleeding. Diclofenac is a popular nonsteroidal anti-inflammatory drug (NSAID) used to treat mild pain.

Take Away Message
- CBD has an excellent safety profile and minor side effects exist only in a minority of users.
- If you take any medication, you should consult with your pharmacist, physician, or other healthcare provider to make sure that CBD does not interfere with the safe blood levels of other medications.

Comparing Apples and Oranges?

Full-spectrum versus isolate

The first issue to address here is whether a full-spectrum "CBD product" (which is actually a "hemp product") or a CBD isolate is better. The answer is simple: it depends on what you are trying to achieve. If you are confused about the source and concentration of CBD and other ingredients, you are not alone. In fact, many CBD users are uncertain as to what kind of CBD to consume.[621]

A CBD full-spectrum product is what it says. It was prepared by conserving multiple compounds found in the hemp plant. A full-spectrum CBD should only contain trace amounts (0.3%) of THC. Because there are different preparation methods and a variety of ways to extract one or more cannabinoid compounds from the plant, the resulting full-spectrum products will differ in their overall content.

Raw full-spectrum is the least processed form, whereas so-called Gold-standard products are further distilled to remove some compounds such as solvents from the mix. Gold-standard full-spectrum products are considered the best form of full-spectrum CBD because they are standardized, which is also why they are typically more expensive. But buyer beware! Since there is currently no good control over the market, anyone can call its products "Gold-standard" without punishment, even if the products are of substandard quality.

Depending on the terpene and/or chlorophyll content, the flavors in full-spectrum products can be somewhat unpleasant. Some manufacturers use the term broad-spectrum CBD for those products that have all THC removed but still contain some of the other cannabinoids in addition to the CBD. It is "buyer beware" again. No standards exist, which is one of the reasons to welcome some form of quality and labeling regulation by the FDA.

Scientifically speaking, CBD isolate is the purest form of CBD you can get. High-quality CBD isolate is typically over 99% pure. In the process of extraction, basically all terpenes and other cannabinoids are removed, and pure CBD is left. You can get CBD isolate either as crystals or as powder. Again, the advantage is that no THC will be in the product, so this form of CBD can be consumed without fear of a positive drug test or experiencing psychotropic effects. CBD isolates could also be recommended to those who want to use higher doses of CBD.

CBD isolates are also somewhat free of heavy flavors, since most of the flavors come from terpenes. On the other hand, valuable compounds, like the terpenes, are taken out during the extraction process, removing the benefits of an "entourage effect" (see next chapter for more detail on this). Many people believe that due to its pure form, CBD isolate might be better to use. However, one study compared full-spectrum CBD with a CBD isolate and found that the full-spectrum CBD was better in preventing inflammation.[622]

In summary, you should decide yourself what form to take depending on your goals. If avoidance of THC and a negative drug test is your goal, you should stick to CBD isolates. If you are not afraid of consuming some THC (remember, some full-spectrum products were measured as having more than the legal limit of THC in them) then you can use full-spectrum CBD. If you prefer isolates but still want the benefits of terpenes and other compounds found in plants, you should consider blending the CBD with plant extracts such as essential oils. More on this topic in Part 3: Combining CBD with Essential Oils.

How to consume CBD

CBD products can be consumed in different ways. As mentioned earlier, they can be eaten as edibles, swallowed as liquids, applied sublingually, vaped, smoked, administered intranasally, applied topically on the skin or into the eye, rectally, or intravenously.

One review looked at the methods of administration in many CBD users and found that most used two different methods. On average, respondents who reported using one method of administration were 1.6 times more likely to use CBD for a medical condition than for general health and well-being. Overall, the most common method reported was the administration of CBD in a sublingual form including liquids administered as sprays, drops, and tinctures. The least common method was topical use.

Medical users reporting one method of administration were 2.4 times more likely to use a topical form, 2.0 times more likely to use an edible form of CBD, and 1.8 times more likely to use CBD in a sublingual or pill or capsule form compared to general health and well-being users.[623] The authors also reported that the preferred method of administration was as follows (in decreasing order): sublingual, vaping, capsules/pills, liquids, smoking, edibles, topical, and others.

Buyers of online CBD products should be aware that more than 20% contained detectable levels of THC when investigated.[624] The same study showed that almost 70% of CBD-labeled products available online may be mislabeled in the sense that 43% of products were under-labeled and 26% were over-labeled for actual CBD content.

In summary, there are multiple ways to consume CBD products. It will very much depend on your preferences and goals which type of consumption/application you select. Of course, you can always combine different methods, like ingesting CBD to get systemic effects such as reduction in overall inflammation and using a topical application to treat local pain. The combination will likely allow you to improve the results.

Different ways to take CBD will also result in different blood levels. High blood levels can be typically achieved by intravenous, intranasal, sublingual, inhalation, and rectal applications. Lower CBD blood levels are typically seen after oral (edibles, liquids, pills, capsules), ophthalmic, and topical applications.

Take Away Message
- Whether a full-spectrum CBD product or a CBD isolate is better depends on what you are trying to achieve.
- If avoidance of THC and a negative drug test is your goal, you should stick to CBD isolates.

- If you are not afraid of consuming some THC, then you can use full-spectrum CBD.
- If you prefer isolates but still want the benefits of terpenes and other compounds found in plants, you should consider blending the CBD with plant extracts such as essential oils.
- There are multiple ways to consume CBD products.
- The effects achieved with CBD will depend on individual factors such as lifestyle, genetics, and overall health, on the CBD type of product you use, on the dose you select, and on the route of administration.

Do You Have an Entourage?

All of you who have been using natural, optimally distilled essential oils have been taking advantage of the entourage effect ever since you started using them. Every essential oil has hundreds of compounds that work together.

Imagine moving into a new place. If you do it alone, as an isolate, there is only that much you can do. You will have trouble lifting heavy furniture like a piano by yourself. But when you surround yourself with a bunch of your best friends who help, the move will be a breeze. That is the entourage effect of your friends. Many film stars surround themselves with an entourage of agents, media managers, assistants, photographer, caterers, and others.

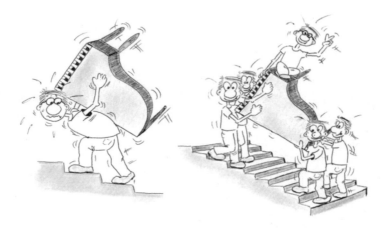

The entourage effect!

C. sativa produces more than 80 terpenophenolic compounds called cannabinoids, which are present in varying relative proportions depending on the strain. [625]

183

Terpenophenolic compounds similar to those produced by *Cannabis* have also been found in plants such as helichrysum.

Terpenoids found in *Cannabis* include β-caryophyllene, carophyllene oxide, myrcene, limonene, linalool, nerolidol, phytol, and alpha-pinene. As mentioned earlier, the sesquiterpene β-caryophyllene is found in many plants.[626] Among those, copaiba is one of the richest in this substance. Other plants containing relatively high levels of β-caryophyllene include black pepper and ylang ylang.

Geranyl pyrophosphate is formed as a precursor in *Cannabis* and is a parent compound to both phytocannabinoids and terpenoids.[627] Terpenoids are pharmacologically versatile: they are lipophilic (they love fat and avoid water) and interact with cell membranes, nerves, muscles, neurotransmitter receptors, G-protein-coupled receptors, second messenger systems, and enzymes.[628]

It is widely believed that terpenes are the basis for the marijuana bud/flower aroma. Over 140 different terpenes have been identified in marijuana.[629] Terpenes are volatile aromatic molecules that evaporate easily. They each have a particular aroma that can be easily picked up by the nose.

Male *Cannabis* plants produce significant amounts of terpenes, the molecules responsible for a plants' individual flavor and scent. Components of marijuana vary depending on whether they have been grown outdoors or indoors. Many terpenoids are Generally Recognized as Safe and are approved by the FDA as food additives.

When researchers compared the results of multiple studies where CBD was given to patients with treatment-resistant seizures, they found that there was a difference in the groups receiving pure CBD isolate versus the ones receiving a full-spectrum CBD product. They concluded that the full-spectrum CBD contained other plant compounds which increased the effect of CBD.

In science, this effect is called the "Entourage Effect." They stated that CBD-rich extracts seem to present a better therapeutic profile than purified CBD, at least in this population of patients with refractory epilepsy.

Patients treated with CBD-rich extracts also reported a lower average dose needed to obtain the desired reduction in seizures compared to those using purified CBD.[630] Similarly, hemp and marijuana plant derivatives with high levels of trans-nerolidol, β-caryophyllene, and d-limonene demonstrated a better entourage effect compared to products containing higher levels of myrcene or terpinolene.[631]

Other studies showed that CBD enriched with other marijuana extracts changed the dose-response curve in patients treated with CBD.[632] So the dose could be lowered to obtain the same results. The effects of anandamide and 2-AG can be enhanced by "entourage compounds" that inhibit their hydrolysis (breakdown), and thereby prolong their action. Such entourage compounds include N-palmitylethanolamide (PEA), N-oleoylethanolamide (SEA), and cis-9-octadecenoamide (OEA, oleamide).[633]

Why would anyone use CBD isolate when the full-spectrum option seems to be better due to its entourage effect? There are a few answers. Full-spectrum is what it says: full-spectrum. It means that is has many compounds in the mix including small amounts of THC. Theoretically, the THC amount should be below 0.3% based on dry weight and not a reason to worry.

However, we know that the amount of each of the compounds in full-spectrum products will vary according to the location and the way hemp plants were grown. The amount of sun light, rain, and other factors will influence the ingredients in a plant. And sometimes parts of the plants that should contain very little THC become contaminated with THC when touching THC-rich parts during harvest or processing.

In addition, there are numerous different types of drug tests, and THC can accumulate in the body due to how much full-spectrum CBD is consumed and for how long. All of this will influence whether traces of THC could potentially be found in a person or not. Research has shown that CBD hemp full-spectrum oil, extracted from hemp plants, may contain enough THC to cause a positive THC/THC metabolite drug test if ingested in very high doses.[634]

The same author concluded that workplace drug testing for cannabinoids remains common yet controversial from a regulatory, political, privacy, medical, and criminal justice viewpoint. He also mentioned that this type of testing is rapidly evolving, with likely expanded regulatory testing of oral fluid and hair and not just urine, each with its own advantages and challenges. The focus on cannabinoid testing appears to be shifting away from marijuana use of any kind at any time (testing urine for an inactive metabolite) into a new direction to enable a decision on whether the person is impaired or not.

This would also make sense in view of the side effects discussed in an earlier chapter. We know that marijuana consumption leads to impairment of cognitive decision-making and more accidents while driving. Therefore, it is illegal, and violators may be charged with driving under the influence. In fact, a study by the Insurance Institute for Highway Safety (IIHS) and Highway Loss Data Institute (HLDI) showed that car crashes are up by as much as 6% in Colorado, Nevada, Oregon, and Washington, states which have legalized the recreational use of marijuana, compared with neighboring states that haven't legalized marijuana for recreational use.[635]

CBD can be transformed to delta-9-tetrahydrocannabinol (THC) and other cannabinoids under acidic conditions. One could argue that when ingested, CBD will be in contact with the acid in our stomach and could potentially be transformed to THC and subsequently show up as a positive drug test.

However, these results seen in the lab seem to not be applicable to real life since the experimental setup cannot mimic the same conditions as found in a human body. The authors note that the conversion of oral CBD to THC and its metabolites has not been observed to occur *in vivo* (in a living human), even after high doses of oral CBD.[636]

The next reason why a CBD isolate may be preferred over a full-spectrum CBD is the confusion regarding the dose of CBD (and other cannabinoids) contained in the blend. It is often very difficult to figure out how much CBD is consumed when taking full-spectrum products. Sometimes the consumer can see the total dose in milligrams of an entire bottle of full-spectrum product and then calculate the amount of CBD per drop or per spray.

However, in many cases the products will have confusing labels, and calculating an exact CBD dose per application is difficult, if not impossible. The use of pure CBD isolate makes it easy to calculate the exact dose per application. When dealing with higher doses, it is especially important to know exactly what is being consumed.

Again, the downside is that we will lose the entourage effect when consuming an isolate. However, there is a solution to this problem: Let's mix the CBD with essential oils! Since natural high-quality essential oils are distilled from plants, they typically contain a full-spectrum of compounds, including terpenoids. If you know what kind of terpenes are found in particular essential oils, you can easily recreate the entourage effect by blending these oils with a CBD isolate and again take advantage of the entourage effect. More to that topic a little later in the book.

Take Away Message
- Every essential oil has hundreds of compounds that work together.
- *C. sativa* produces more than 80 terpenophenolic compounds.
- β-caryophyllene is a terpenoid found in *Cannabis* as well as many other plants.

- Terpenes are probably the basis for the marijuana bud/flower aroma.
- Full-spectrum CBD has the entourage effect, meaning that additional plant compounds increase the benefits.
- But full-spectrum products increase the risk of THC entering the body.
- It is often very difficult to figure out how much CBD is consumed when taking full-spectrum products.
- The downside is that we will lose the entourage effect when consuming an isolate.
- Recreate the entourage effect by blending specific oils, and their terpenes, with a CBD isolate.

How Much CBD Should You Take?

Many CBD beginners will be completely lost as to how much CBD to consume. I already mentioned earlier that the route of administration is important with regards to absorption and bioavailability. But just as significant are the formulation and supplementation of additives such as simple oils to enhance both the absorption and bioavailability of the product.

Many manufacturers do a poor job in telling the buyer exactly how much CBD is contained in the product. There are many reasons for that. One of them has to do with the changing laws and the uncertainty associated with CBD. Some manufacturers elect to not mention CBD at all on their labels in order to avoid attention of the various state agencies. Others are simply doing a lousy job in calculating an exact dose.

In 2017, one study found that basically 70% of CBD products tested in their lab had higher or lower concentrations of CBD compared to what was declared on the label. To be precise, 43% of products were under-labeled, 26% were over-labeled, and only 31% were accurately labeled.[637]

At a public FDA hearing in May 2019, pharmacists reported that while measuring CBD content in commercially available products, the amount of CBD was misrepresented in most labels. Some products contained no CBD at all, while others had 23 times more than declared on the label.

It is also very worrisome that several products had more than the 0.3% legally permitted THC in the full-spectrum oil. One of the products investigated contained a whopping 45% THC.[638]

Such problems in the market make a strong argument for better supervision and regulations. Therefore, the FDA statements regarding the oversight of CBD products have some validity.

Let's look at some clinical studies with humans to see what kind of dosing ranges they used and whether those amounts of CBD were safe and well tolerated. A recent study evaluated the safety of increasing CBD administration to healthy volunteers.[639]

The doses used were 1500, 3000, 4500, or 6000mg CBD when using single daily doses and 750 or 1500mg CBD when using two doses per day. This was compared to both placebo and high-fat food groups. After single oral doses, CBD appeared rapidly in plasma and time to maximum blood concentration was approximately four to five hours.

CBD reached steady state in blood levels after approximately two days. A high-fat meal increased CBD blood levels. In fact, the amount of CBD actually available for the body was four to five times higher when taken with fat such as oils. This supports the practice of blending CBD with an oil like olive, hemp, sesame, flax seed, and avocado, or essential oils.

Terminal elimination half-life was approximately 60 hours after 750 and 1500mg CBD twice daily, and effective half-life for all doses ranged from 10 to 17 hours. Terminal plasma half-life is the time required to divide the plasma (blood) concentration by two after reaching pseudo-equilibrium, whereas effective half-life describes the time required to eliminate half of a single administered dose.[640] The terminal half-life is especially relevant to multiple dosing regimens, because it controls for the degree of drug accumulation, concentration fluctuations, and the time taken to reach equilibrium.

Diarrhea, nausea, headache, and somnolence (drowsiness) were the most common adverse events. The authors concluded that administration, either as single or multiple dose regimen with total doses up to 6000mg CBD daily, was safe and well tolerated. Side effects were mild to moderate. and no participant quit the study due to side effects.

Chronic use and high doses of up to 1500mg per day have been repeatedly shown to be well tolerated by humans.[641] CBD, at an average daily dose of about 700mg/day for 6 weeks, was neither symptomatically effective nor toxic, relative to a placebo, in a study involving patients with the neurological condition Huntington's disease.[642] Another study used coadministration of CBD and fentanyl (a potent opioid). The results showed that CBD does not exacerbate adverse effects associated with intravenous fentanyl administration. The authors concluded that coadministration of CBD and opioids was safe and well tolerated.[643]

One patient with dystonic disorder (dystonia is a movement disorder in which a person's muscles contract uncontrollably) was chronically treated with 600mg daily oral doses of CBD and no problems were reported. His urine was analyzed to get a better understanding about metabolism of CBD.[644]

One study asked the question whether pretreatment with 600mg CBD and subsequent THC administration could reduce THC's psychotic and anxiety symptoms.[645] The results showed CBD's ability to block the psychotogenic effects of THC. In addition, no effects on peripheral cardiovascular measures such as heart rate and blood pressure were measured at this dose.

Another study used 600mg CBD on 16 healthy non-anxious subjects and found no differences in heart rate and blood pressure between the CBD and placebo groups.[646] One case report describes a patient treated for marijuana withdrawal according to the following oral CBD regimen: 300mg on Day 1, 600mg on Days 2–10, and 300mg on Day 11. The CBD treatment resulted in a fast and progressive reduction in the withdrawal, dissociative, and anxiety symptoms associated with marijuana abuse.[647]

One study conducted on 225 pediatric patients with Lennox-Gastaut Syndrome (a rare form of epilepsy) used CBD (either 10mg/kg body weight or 20mg/kg body weight) administered by two doses daily for 14 weeks.[648] The average age of the children was 13 years old. A normal weight of a 13-year-old is around 45 kg. This means that the children received around 450 or 900mg of CBD per day depending on the study group. The CBD was administered in addition to their regular anti-seizure medication.

The decrease in seizure frequency during the treatment period was 41.9% in the 20mg/kg CBD group, 37.2% in the 10mg/kg CBD group, and 17.2% in the placebo group. The most common adverse events among the patients in the CBD groups were somnolence, decreased appetite, and diarrhea. These events occurred more frequently in the higher dose group. Overall, CBD administration was safe and the described side effects were minor to moderate.

Another very similar study used only 20mg/kg body weight CBD and placebo for 14 weeks. This study included 171 patients with Lennox-Gastaut Syndrome as well.[649] Reduction in monthly seizure frequency from baseline was 43.9% in the CBD group and 21.8% in the placebo group. The most common adverse events were diarrhea, somnolence, pyrexia (fever), decreased appetite, and vomiting. 14% of patients in the CBD group and 1% of patients in the placebo group withdrew from the study because of these adverse events.

Another study addressing fear of public speaking used 600mg CBD per day without problems.[650] Overall, CBD dosing in a variety of clinical trials in humans ranges from 20mg to 6000mg per day.

Most therapeutic applications of CBD in non-healthy volunteers use CBD in the range of 300 to 1500mg per day. Many authors suggest that CBD for wellness and overall health should be started at doses around 10 to 20mg per day and then doubled every three to five days until the desired effect is reached.

Since many people will not feel a short-term difference when using CBD for wellness purposes (after all, CBD has no psychotic effects such as making you high), it could be argued that the daily dose should be below what is used in clinical trials to treat disease. In other words, a daily dose of 10 to 300mg per day should likely be enough to improve overall health.

It is my personal experience that doses between 100 to 300mg are sufficient to feel some of the beneficial effects like increased comfort in joints and muscles, deep sleep, and a healthy immune system. Long-term effects would likely be better bones, cardiovascular performance, sleep, immune system, and cognitive function. When using CBD for specific health problems the daily dose could go up to around 750mg based on these studies. In either case, it is good to know that doses up to 6000mg per day have shown to be safe.

In summary, the best suggestion for people new to CBD is to have them start low at 10 to 20mg per day and then slowly increase the dose until they feel a beneficial effect. That will likely happen around 50 to 200mg unless they are trying to treat a more serious condition. In that case, doses between 100 and 750mg might be needed. Most clinical trials using CBD on sick patients have been using doses of 500mg per day and higher. There is also the fact that CBD found in "Gold Standard" products might be stronger than raw CBD products. And because manufactures can currently name their products as they wish, it is again buyer beware.

Please remember that each person will act differently to various doses of CBD. The reason for this is that each person has a different lifestyle which leads to a different amount of ECS receptors. We all eat and exercise differently and have distinct genetics. I also strongly believe that the quantity of toxic compounds in one's life, such as personal care products, household cleaners, soaps and shampoos, laundry detergents, and so on, plays a major role in our overall health and in the manner CBD may act in our body.

Take Away Message
- Many manufacturers do a poor job in telling the buyer exactly how much CBD is contained in the product.
- Overall, CBD dosing in a variety of clinical trials in humans ranges from 20mg to 6000mg per day.
- The best suggestion for people new to CBD is to start low at 10 to 20mg per day and then slowly increase until they feel a beneficial effect.
- A daily dose of 10 to 300mg per day should be enough to improve overall health.
- 100 to 300mg of CBD per day should be enough to treat mild to moderate conditions.
- Please remember that each person will act differently to various doses of CBD.

CBD for Animals

CBD has become popular among animal lovers, and many companies now offer CBD products for pets. As I am not a licensed veterinarian, I will not make any suggestions as to which conditions can be treated with what doses in different animal species. However, I will mention a few studies to give you an idea of what has been done in veterinary science. Due to the myriad of laws concerning *Cannabis*-derived products, there is little empirical research regarding the veterinary use of CBD.

The very first animal studies with marijuana-based products as an anti-seizure medication were published in 1843 by W.B. O'Shaughnessy.[651] After testing the behavioral effects of various preparations of *Cannabis indica* in healthy fish, dogs, swine, vultures, crows, horses, deer, monkeys, goats, sheep, and cows, he went on to test these products in humans. Little is known on what exactly he used, how much of it, and how he administered it.

A recent review conducted via the Veterinary Information Network looked at 2,130 returned questionnaires.[652] The results showed that 61.5% of veterinarians felt comfortable discussing the use of CBD with their colleagues, but only 45.5% felt comfortable discussing this topic with clients. No differences were found based on the state of practice, but recent graduates were less comfortable discussing the topic. Overall, CBD was most frequently discussed as a potential treatment for pain management, anxiety, and seizures.

Veterinarians practicing in states with legalized recreational marijuana were more likely to recommend the use of CBD. Recent veterinary graduates were less likely to recommend or prescribe CBD. The most commonly used CBD formulations were oil/extract and edibles. The participants also felt their state veterinary associations and veterinary boards did not provide sufficient guidance for them to practice within applicable laws. And finally, most veterinarians expressed support for use of CBD products for animals.

One study used two different doses of CBD enriched oil, namely two and eight mg per kg body weight to treat osteoarthritis in dogs.[653] This would translate to a total CBD dose of 10 to 40mg for small dogs, 30 to 120mg for medium size dogs, and 50 to 200mg for large dogs. Pharmacokinetics revealed an elimination half-life of 4.2 hours at both doses and no observable side effects. Veterinary assessment showed significantly decreased pain during the time of CBD treatment. The authors concluded that a dose of two mg per kg twice a day would be appropriate in this setting.

Another study with dogs found that bioavailability after oral administration of 180mg ranged from zero to 19%.[654] The results of this study show that similarly to humans, CBD is not well-absorbed in dogs after oral administration. This low bioavailability is likely due to the first pass effect in the liver as described earlier. The intravenous application of 45 and 90mg showed that the CBD was rapidly distributed, and the terminal half-life was 9 hours.

Other veterinarians suggested that oral dosing of CBD in dogs and cats is 0.02 mg/kg to 0.1 mg/kg given twice daily. According to one veterinarian, most dogs do well at 0.05 mg/kg twice daily for pain management, while cats do well at 0.025 mg/kg twice daily.[655] This would translate to doses of about 0.5 to 2.5mg CBD for dogs and half of that for cats.

Preliminary data of another study showed that 89% of dogs who received CBD in a clinical trial had a reduction in the frequency of seizures.[656] The American Kennel Club Canine Health Foundation also reported that new studies to investigate the use of CBD in dogs with therapy-resistant epilepsy are ongoing.[657]

In summary, clinical studies evaluating the use of either marijuana or CBD alone in animals are lacking. Despite the lack of evidence, many companies are now selling CBD products for pets. Since animals likely have a very similar ECS compared to humans, it makes sense that CBD can be used for animals. However, I will leave the choice of whether to use CBD for your pets to you and your veterinarian.

Take Away Message
- Due to the myriad of laws concerning *Cannabis*-derived products, there is little empirical research regarding the veterinary use of CBD.
- The very first animal studies with marijuana-based products as an anti-seizure medication were published in 1843 by W.B. O'Shaughnessy.
- Overall, CBD was most frequently discussed as a potential treatment for pain management, anxiety, and seizures in animals.

Part 3: Combining CBD with EOs

CBD and Essential Oils

Before we dive into this intriguing topic, I must mention that the research of CBD combined with essential oils is in its infancy and very little can be found in medical and scientific literature. Much more has been written about hemp and marijuana and how they can influence the endocannabinoid system. Just because a plant itself exerts beneficial effects on this system, it does not automatically mean that an essential oil of that same plant has the same or even a similar effect.

Often, during the process of distillation, certain plant compounds get lost or changed by the heat of the steam and don't make it into the final essential oil product. On the other hand, essential oils are known to be very powerful since they are highly concentrated. With that in mind, we must be careful not to make wrong assumptions.

However, since essential oils are in general very safe, especially those labelled as dietary supplements, I encourage you to start experimenting with them after you read this chapter. Be aware, though, that the quality of essential oils used is extremely important. There is no point in blending a high-quality CBD isolate with substandard and cheap essential oils, which are likely adulterated with synthetics and contaminated with toxins.

Just like when choosing a CBD isolate option, it is necessary to look for the same Seed to Seal quality standards for the essential oils. They should be 100% pure and therapeutic grade. A high-quality essential oil company will have full transparency regarding the source of the plants, including farms that are open to the public and easily visited.

The following list of essential oils is certainly not exhaustive since many more essential oils are currently on the market. They however represent some of the essential oils I have been experimenting with by combining them with CBD. Feel free to do your own research, let your innovative juices flow, and then make your own creations.

For this section, first I will present a brief summary of the literature on some of the essential oils I have been using together with CBD, and then I will explain what I have been mixing for my personal use.

Disclaimer: This book is based on the author's personal knowledge and experience. It is well known that different people react differently when it comes to natural substances and especially the endocannabinoid system. The information provided in this book is for informational purposes only and is not intended to replace any medical advice or to halt proper medical treatment. Please consult with your physician and healthcare provider if you have any medical condition or if you are pregnant. The information in this book, and especially the following chapters, is for educational purposes only.

Many of the following suggestions are not based on scientific data simply because very little exists on the combination of CBD with essential oils or other type of natural products. It has also been mentioned earlier that only high-quality, heavy-metal and toxin-free products should be used for both CBD and essential oils.

Some remarks regarding compliant statements and health claims for natural products: Many essential oils have by now been labeled as dietary supplements. When we discuss dietary supplements, we can cite references and summarize or present results from scientific studies.

I have not mentioned any specific brand of CBD or essential oils despite having some clear preferences. I have avoided to name specific brands on purpose. This book was not written as advertisement for specific products but rather as an educational tool for everyone. However, if you currently do not have any guidance on essential oils or CBD brands, use the contact information at the end of the book to learn more about my choices of CBD and essential oils.

Throughout the book I take advantage of the rules which allow me to quote and list scientific research and refer to the sources of these quotes. So, there will be information on the medical benefits of either CBD, essential oils, or other treasures of nature in conjunction with the mentioning of health conditions.

The studies discussed with each of the essential oils only represents a fraction of what has been published. Those selected here are just to show you what intrigued me to use these oils together with CBD. And as mentioned before, the addition of essential oils to CBD allows for a re-creation of the entourage effect, which was lost when isolating pure CBD crystals from the full-spectrum plant material.

The Food and Drug Administration (FDA) has not evaluated or approved the various statements made in this book. The combinations of CBD and essential oils, or other plants mentioned in the next chapters, are not intended to prevent, diagnose, treat or cure any disease condition but rather to support the readers in their quest for wellness and health.

Copaiba

One huge question is whether copaiba and CBD are the same. Many believe that we could replace CBD by simply using the essential oil of the copaiba tree. Is that true? Let's have a closer look at this plant.

Amazonian medical practitioners have been using copaiba for a long time because of its anti-inflammatory and wound healing effects. Copaiba resin was first described as "Copei" in a report by Petrus Martys to Pope Leo X published by Herr in Strasburg in 1534.[658] About a century later in 1625, the Portuguese monk Manuel Tristaon described the wound healing effects of copaiba which he called "cupayba." This medicinal compound was then brought back from the New World by the Jesuits. This is the reason why it is also known as Jesuit's balsam.[659]

The tree itself was first described by Marcgraf and Piso in 1638, who employed the name "copaiba" without designating the species. There are more than 70 *Copaifera* species distributed throughout the world, and Brazil is the country with the greatest biodiversity of *Copaifera* with 26 species and eight varieties.[660] Today, Brazil produces approximately 95% of this oil-resin, exporting more than 500 tons each year.[661] Copaiba resin is obtained by drilling holes in the tree trunk, with each yielding up to 12 gallons.

Both copaiba and *Cannabis* contain significant amounts of β-caryophyllene (BCP). BCP is a sesquiterpene found in many plants and is an FDA approved food additive. Chromatographic studies showed that three different varieties of Copaiba contained up to 58% β-caryophyllene (58, 41, and 20%, respectively), followed by alpha-humulene, alpha-copaene, alpha-bergamotene, alpha-pinene, and delta-cadinene.[662] This compares to the BCP found in cannabinoids of up to 35%.[663]

Other plants containing BCP include black pepper (30%), ylang ylang (19%), melissa (16%), lavandin (10%), clove (8%), Roman chamomile (8%), frankincense (6%), yarrow (6%), carrot seed (5%), cinnamon bark (5%), lavender (5%), lemongrass (5%), thyme (5%), savory (5%), sage (5%), oregano (5%), rosemary (2%), and hops.[664,665,666] In fact, almost 18% of all known essential oils contain 5% or more BCP.[667]

Similar to CBD, BCP selectively binds to CB2 receptors and is therefore a functional non-psychoactive anti-inflammatory CB2 receptor ligand.[668] Orally administered β-caryophyllene produces strong CB2-dependent anti-inflammatory and analgesic effects.[669] One study described how effective it is at reducing neuropathic pain.[670] Other researchers found it to be a good treatment modality for chronic pain.[671]

Positive effects could be found in Parkinson's patients where BCP displayed neuroprotective action via activation of CB2 receptors.[672] Benefits could also be shown in arthritis and cancer patients.[673,674] It is well established that copaiba oil with its high BCP content exerts anti-inflammatory effects while being well tolerated.[675] Non-essential oil users also enjoy these benefits, as most people get BCP from the ingestion of vegetables. This is one the ways through which vegetables exert anti-inflammatory effects in the human body.

Medical literature on copaiba essential oil is also impressive. Studies described it to have neuroprotective[676], anxiolytic[677], antioxidant, anti-inflammatory[678], and anti-arthritic[679] benefits.

The mechanism of action is not necessarily the same because CBD may work via influencing the availability of the endocannabinoid anandamide whereas BCP from copaiba and *Cannabis* can selectively bind to CB2 receptors. One could speculate that BCP elicits a higher response from CB receptors than CBD, since CBD has more of a balancing role on the endocannabinoid system and can also dampen overactivity of CB receptors by regulating our own endocannabinoids.

So, are copaiba and CBD the same? No, however both plant extracts contain BCP and could therefore go well together. If you simply want to have a high intake of BCP you could either use copaiba alone, or in combination with CBD, or in combination with many other essential oils and vegetables. Both CBD, whether as an isolate or as a full-spectrum product containing many more compounds including BCP, and copaiba, due to its significant amounts of BCP, will influence CB receptors, particularly the CB2 type.

Several studies show that the effects of CBD and copaiba seem to be very comparable on neuroprotection, pain reduction, anti-inflammatory actions, support in autoimmune diseases like multiple sclerosis, as well as benefiting patients with neurological diseases and cancer.

As mentioned earlier, copaiba also contains other very important compounds besides BCP. These compounds could be partially responsible for the beneficial effects of copaiba. All in all, copaiba essential oil is certainly a very interesting essential oil to combine with CBD, and perhaps the combination of the two enhances the effects of each.

Lavender

Lavender is one of the most popular essential oils. It has been used for centuries because of its calming, sleep benefiting, and skin-supporting properties. But lavender has many other uses and properties, and research has a large body of literature on this essential oil. One scientific review mentions the benefits of lavender with its anxiolytic, mood stabilizer, sedative, analgesic, anticonvulsive, and neuroprotective properties.[680]

Sleep: Several studies have been published on this topic. One found that the sleep quality of 158 women in the postpartum period was significantly different between the control (no lavender inhalation) and inhalation of lavender essential oil groups. They saw improved sleep after 8 weeks when taking 10 deep breaths of lavender scent 4 times a week. They concluded that lavender aromatherapy was effective in the improvement of mothers' sleep quality.[681]

Another interesting study looked at the consumption of lavender tea by postpartum mothers and realized that lavender made the mothers perceive less fatigue and less depression while showing greater bonding with their infant.[682]

Yet another study investigated the sleep quality of college students via Fitbit devices and found that lavender inhaled via an inhalation patch applied to their chest combined with better sleep hygiene (common measures to improve sleep), and sleep hygiene alone to a lesser degree, improved sleep quality.[683] A study with 42 female college students in Korea suffering from insomnia found that lavender aromatherapy had a beneficial effect on insomnia and depression.[684]

Another study looked at 70 chemotherapy patients and discovered that anxiety values before and after chemotherapy were significantly different. Those who were smelling lavender were much more relaxed. In addition, a significant positive change in sleep quality before and after chemotherapy was also observed.[685] Similar results were obtained in a study investigating hemodialysis patients. The scientists found that daytime sleepiness declined, and nightly sleep duration increased in the group using lavender inhalation.[686]

Anxiety: Lavender essential oil is used and approved by the European Medicines Agency as herbal medicine to relieve stress and anxiety.[687] Studies demonstrated that lavender essential oil, and its two primary terpenoid constituents linalool and linalyl acetate, elicit an anxiolytic effect in combination with reduction of 5HT1A receptor activity.[688]

Lavender essential oil also works by reducing the calcium influx into cells, leading to reduced brainwave activity at higher frequencies.[689] We also know from a variety of studies that lavender essential oil influences different receptors in the brain either directly by binding to them or indirectly by influencing other receptors first.

My own studies using quantitative EEG analysis showed complete calming of the entire limbic system including the hippocampus after just three seconds of inhalation of lavender essential oil. The same results were also obtained with inhalation of frankincense and a blend containing lavender, cedarwood, lime, ocotea, and copaiba essential oils as well as vanilla extract. The actual video recording of that personal study was shown in the movie *Ancient Secrets of Essential Oils* and in several of the educational video collections of the Global Online Essential Oils Symposium published by my team, BioCode Academy.[690]

Hair: One study showed that the topical application of lavender essential oil had a marked hair growth-promoting effect, as observed morphologically and histologically. After only four weeks, the measurements showed a significantly increased number of hair follicles, deepened hair follicle depth, and a thickened dermal layer.[691] In fact, the use of lavender resulted in better hair growth compared to the topical application of the commonly used prescription medication.

No side effects were observed with the lavender application, in contrast to the group using the prescription medication. Another finding was that mast cells were significantly reduced in the lavender group. Mast cells are part of the immune cells and are lower if there is a reduction in inflammation. Another study using peppermint essential oil had similar results (*see Peppermint*).

Pain: Lavender has excellent and well-documented pain-relieving properties. One study with migraine patients demonstrated that lavender essential oil inhalation benefited most of the patients. From 129 headache attacks, 92 responded entirely or partially to lavender. The percentage of responders was significantly higher in the lavender inhalation group than the placebo group.[692] Several studies found that aromatherapy massage with lavender essential oil was effective in relieving pain in patients with knee osteoarthritis, and that this led to immediate increase in daily activities for four weeks.[693,694]

Wound healing: Several authors mention the benefits lavender can have on wound healing.[695] In a study investigating wound healing from recurrent aphthous ulceration (canker sores in the mouth), patients treated topically with lavender oil showed a significant reduction in inflammation level, ulcer size, healing time, and pain relief mostly from the first dose, compared to the baseline and placebo.[696] It is also interesting to note that no side effects were reported.

Another study demonstrated that the topical application of lavender essential oil promoted collagen synthesis and differentiation of fibroblasts (cells needed for wound healing), accompanied by up-regulation of TGF-β (a protein needed for control of cell growth). These data suggest that lavender oil promotes the early phase of wound healing by accelerating the formation of granulation tissue, by tissue remodeling, by collagen replacement, and by wound contraction through up-regulation of TGF-β.[697]

Topical application of lavender essential oil demonstrated better results compared with regular treatment in regards to pain, redness, swelling, and wound healing in 60 women five days after an episiotomy, a surgical cut made at the opening of the vagina during childbirth to facilitate the birth of the baby.[698] Another study showed that inhalation of lavender essential oil also decreased menstruation pain in 200 women when inhaled for about 30 minutes during the first three days of the cycle.[699] It took two full menstruation cycles to see these effects in this particular study.

It is very interesting that CBD also binds to some of the exact same receptors as lavender, and the intake of CBD also results in reduced anxiety, improved sleep, reduced pain, and potentially improved early phase wound healing through reduction of inflammation. All of these facts intrigued me, and now I often combine CBD with lavender essential oil.

Peppermint

Peppermint is well known for its beneficial effects on humans. Mint has been used for health purposes for several thousand years. Its use was recorded in Ancient Greece, Rome, and Egypt. However, peppermint was not recognized as a distinct kind of mint until the 1700s.[700] Peppermint is mostly used in folk medicine for its benefits during breathing problems, as seen with the common cold, digestive problems, such as nausea, vomiting, and irritable bowel syndrome (IBS), and headaches or other painful conditions.

Improved Breathing, Oxygenation, and Athletic Performance: One study found the that the ingestion of a very small amount (0.05ml ~ one drop) of peppermint essential oil significantly improved lung and breathing function as measured by spirometric tests (lung function tests).[701] The authors concluded that these benefits were likely due to the peppermint effects on the small airways of the lung.

Peppermint essential oil relaxed the muscles around the small airways while not affecting the surface of the tiny bubbles in the lungs, the alveoli, where the gas exchange takes place. In addition to improved lung function, the study also demonstrated a significant increase in grip force (36.1%), standing vertical jump (7.0%), and standing long jump (6.4%).

Another similar study had 12 healthy volunteers consume one drop of peppermint essential oil in their drinks and found the same effects. After ten days, the authors not only found a significant improvement in lung function tests but also a significant improvement in athletic performance. There was a longer time until exhaustion while exercising and increased power during the exercise.[702] In addition, they found that both resting and exercise heart rates were significantly decreased after ten days. Similarly, the chest circumference during maximum exhale and blood pressure significantly decreased in the same time period.

212

Nausea and Vomiting: 5-HT3 receptors found in the vagus nerve and some areas of the brain are a very specific subtype of the serotonin receptor family. The highest concentration of the receptors is found in the brainstem where they play an important role in nausea and emesis (vomiting).[703] Of course the same receptors are found in the enteric nervous system (nerves of the gut).

Menthol from peppermint acts as an antagonist for 5-HT3 and can therefore reduce nausea and vomiting.[704] The same was shown for CBD and our own endocannabinoid anandamide.[705,706] So, both CBD and menthol have anti-nausea and anti-emetic effects. Antagonists of the 5-HT3 receptor are currently one of the most effective therapeutic agents in treatment of chemotherapy-induced nausea, vomiting, and irritable bowel syndrome.

A study with 35 women recovering from C-sections showed that postoperative nausea and vomiting was significantly reduced after peppermint inhalation, much more compared to both the placebo group that used water and the medical treatment group that got anti-nausea medication.[707] Peppermint essential oil inhalation also significantly decreased nausea in heart surgery patients after only two minutes.[708] However, two studies with pregnant women did not find a difference when using peppermint aromatherapy.[709,710]

An older study also found peppermint essential oil inhalation effective in the postoperative setting and calculated a cost of about 50 cents to one dollar per patient, significantly less than the costs of a traditional antiemetic drug.[711] And finally, a review of several articles using peppermint against nausea and vomiting concluded that the inhaled vapor of peppermint or ginger essential oils not only reduced the incidence and severity of nausea and vomiting, but also decreased anti-emetic medication requirements, consequently improving patient satisfaction.[712]

Hair Growth: One study found that the topical application of peppermint essential oil significantly increased dermal thickness of the scalp, the hair follicle number, and the hair follicle depth.[713] Genes responsible for hair growth were also activated, and the treatment was safe and showed no adverse effects.

Similar results were obtained with rosemary, cedarwood, thyme, and lavender essential oils.[714] Sometimes, hair loss is caused by inflammatory conditions. We know that CBD has excellent anti-inflammatory properties and combining it with the topical application of these essential oils could be very interesting, however the scientific community has not yet reached a conclusion on whether CBD is beneficial for hair growth or not.

Cognitive Function: The freshness of peppermint scent has also been associated with improved cognitive performance. One study with 140 volunteers demonstrated that inhalation of peppermint was able to enhance memory.[715] It also resulted in a decrease of daytime sleepiness,[716] and another study showed that peppermint odor improved cognitive processing.[717] One group of researchers demonstrated nicely that scents of peppermint and cinnamon increased attention in drivers.[718]

In my own research using quantitative EEG, I found that the inhalation of peppermint essential oil increased the activity of beta frequency waves in the left frontal part of my brain after about three to five seconds. This result indicates increased attention and information intake for further processing by the brain.

Perception of Cold Temperatures: TRPM8 and TRPA1 receptors are involved in feeling cold sensations. They are both from the transient receptor potential (TRP) family of receptors. Interestingly, TRPM8 is activated by menthol, so it is called the menthol receptor, and peppermint essential oil contains up to 44% menthol.[719]

Activation of this receptor is one of the mechanisms by which we humans perceive cold temperatures.[720] The same authors found that the other receptor, TRPA1, can be activated by the pungent ingredients in mustard and the constituents found in cinnamon, both of which also lead to cold perception.

What makes this so interesting is the fact that CBD, other cannabinoids, and the entire ECS is involved in thermoregulation of the body. It is now known that both CBD and THC also interact with TRP receptors.[721] It seems that CBD in fact is an antagonist for the TRPM8 receptor and inhibits some of the cold sensation.[722] This makes sense in the context of balancing the cold/heat thermoregulation within our body. Again, it seems that CBD can help maintain homeostasis by inhibiting overstimulation of cold receptors.

It seems that peppermint and CBD interact with a variety of the same receptors in our body. Sometimes they have the same effect and sometimes they do the opposite. Peppermint essential oil also contains a small amount of BCP (about 1%) which by itself binds to CB receptors. The combination of CBD with peppermint essential oils is certainly intriguing when it comes to nausea, vomiting, or other digestive problems. Both have an excellent safety profile and should therefore not cause major problems when taken internally.

And the addition of peppermint, or other delicious essential oils, to pure CBD isolates or even to full-spectrum CBD, could enhance the flavor profile of the products.

Frankincense

Boswellia resin, also called frankincense or olibanum, has been used as incense in religious and cultural ceremonies since the beginning of written history. In medicine, it has also been used for centuries. Research results showed benefits in treatment of inflammatory conditions, microbial infections, depressions, pain, cancerous diseases, as well as wound healing.[723,724,725,726,727] This and the fact that we have many published articles in the medical literature showing the benefits of frankincense makes this essential oil a very interesting natural substance to work with.

Pain: Topical application of frankincense essential oil or its active ingredients (including α-pinene, linalool, and 1-octanol) exhibit significantly anti-inflammatory and analgesic (pain-reducing) effects.[728] Frankincense also demonstrated significant anti-inflammatory and analgesic activities in combination with myrrh.[729]

One study with 12 healthy volunteers demonstrated that frankincense significantly increased the pain threshold and pain tolerance compared to a placebo.[730] In another study with 30 patients suffering from osteoarthritis, all patients receiving frankincense reported a decrease in knee pain, increase in knee flexion, decrease in swelling in the knee joint, and increase in walking distance. The authors recommended using frankincense not only for these patients but also for those with other forms of arthritis.[731]

Some authors suggested that frankincense represents a promising alternative to non-steroidal anti-inflammatory drugs (NSAIDs), because it has good analgesic properties but none of the downsides of NSAIDs like gastrointestinal or cardiovascular adverse effects.[732] Another study with patients suffering from chronic cluster headaches, including sleep disturbances, demonstrated that frankincense treatment resulted in a rapid and long-lasting reduction of the intensity and frequency of headaches.[733] The pain-relieving properties of frankincense are well documented.

Anxiety and Depression: Incensole acetate (IA), a frankincense resin constituent, is a potent agonist for the transient receptor potential vanillin (TRPV3) and causes anxiolytic-like and anti-depressive effects.[734]

In my own quantitative EEG studies, frankincense immediately calmed the entire limbic system indicating a rapid onset of anxiolytic effects.

Another study showed that IA from frankincense modulates the hypothalamic-pituitary-adrenal (HPA) axis and influences hippocampal gene expression, leading to beneficial behavioral effects. This makes it a novel natural treatment of depressive-like disorders.[735] The anxiolytic and anti-depressive effects might be the reasons why frankincense has been burned as incense for centuries.[736]

Cancer: There is a large body of literature describing the benefits of frankincense and frankincense essential oil against cancer. One study demonstrated that sacred frankincense (*Boswellia sacra*) essential oil induced breast cancer cell-specific cytotoxicity (destroying cancer cells) in advanced breast cancer.[737] 3-O-acetyl-11-keto-β-boswellic acid from the gum resin from frankincense (*Boswellia serrata*) also has pronounced and irreversible inhibitory effects on human leukemia cells.[738]

A case report described the anti-cancer effects of frankincense in a patient with urogenital cancer.[739] Other studies demonstrated a significant reduction in brain cancer tumor volume after treatment with frankincense.[740] Another case report showed that multiple brain metastases were successfully reversed using frankincense in a breast cancer patient who had not shown improvement after standard therapy.[741]

The frankincense terpenoid acetyl-11-keto-β-boswellic acid is a potent anti-proliferative (prevents growth of cancer cells) and apoptotic (lets cancer cells commit suicide) agent and significantly inhibits both the survival of glioblastoma cancer cells in vitro and the growth of tumors generated by these cells.[742] Another study confirmed the anti-cancer activity of frankincense in five leukemia and two brain cancer cell lines.[743]

Despite the large body of scientific evidence with regards to using frankincense against various forms of cancer, the majority of these studies are either cell line or animal studies. Human studies are mostly case reports. Large well-designed randomized clinic trials using frankincense and frankincense essential oil against cancer are missing.

As mentioned, frankincense contains IA which binds as a potent agonist to transient receptor potential vanillin (TRPV) receptors. Interestingly, CBD has also shown to bind to these receptors. Frankincense also contains up to 8% of BCP depending on the species of *Boswellia*. All of that could explain the similar beneficial effects of CBD and frankincense on pain, anxiety, depression, and cancer.

Citrus Fruits

Citrus fruit cultivation goes way back in time, and the consumption of various citrus fruits like lemon, orange, tangerine, yuzu, bergamot, lime, mandarin, and others for their health benefits and taste is well-known. About 50% of a citrus fruit is considered waste product and, in most cases, only the inner part of the fresh fruit is used for consumption as food or beverage. It is also rich in vitamin C, an important antioxidant.

The "waste" is comprised of the pulp, peel, seeds, and fibers of the fruit, and contains very important compounds such as d-limonene, flavonoids, carotenoids, dietary fibers, soluble sugars, cellulose, hemicellulose, pectin, polyphenols, ascorbic acid, and essential oils. [744]

Limonene is a terpene found in citrus fruits, but it is also found in the *Cannabis* plant, vegetables (especially carrots), coffee, beverages, meat, and spices (like nutmeg, for example).[745,746] Sweet orange, bitter orange, tangerine, mandarin, and grapefruit essential oils contain anywhere from 65 to 96% d-limonene (an isomer, or special chemical structure, of limonene).[747]

The biological activities of d-limonene have been well described in literature. D-limonene is known to exhibit potent anti-cancer,[748] anxiolytic,[749] anti-inflammatory,[750] antioxidant, liver-protecting, blood pressure-reducing,[751] cholesterol-lowering,[752] and immune-stimulating properties in humans.[753] One study researched the effects of d-limonene after a one-week treatment.

The authors concluded that significant changes occurred on a variety of receptors, such as GABA, 5-hydroxyindoleacetic acid (5-HIAA) and 5-HT (family of serotonin receptors).[754] This is important because it can explain the anxiolytic and stress-reducing effects of aromatherapy with essential oils from citrus fruits, but it also shows the similarity of the effects of CBD and citrus fruits when it comes to the activation of certain receptors in the brain.

Another study demonstrated the sedative effects of limonene and concluded that the mechanism was the regulation of dopamine levels (one of our neurotransmitters) and the activation of the 5-HT receptor function.[755] This was confirmed by another study using lemon essential oil. The anxiolytic-like activity observed after acute and 14-day repeated dosing was also mediated by the serotonergic system, i.e. activation of 5-HT1A serotonin receptors.[756]

One study demonstrated that the pleasant odor of limonene alone can have a positive effect on mood.[757] Another study found that aromatherapy with orange essential oil in the waiting room of a dentist's office could reduce the anxiety, and improve the mood, of female patients.[758] Orange aromatherapy also demonstrated a reduction of patient anxiety before and after dental surgery.[759]

Other studies demonstrate the benefits of limonene in stroke-associated cerebral and vascular damage under conditions of hypertension.[760] Citrus fruits and their components, like flavonoids and monoterpenes, exhibit a remarkable spectrum of effective biological activities, particularly in anti-tumorigenesis (prevention of growth of cancers).[761,762]

One review and analysis of multiple articles writing about this topic found an inverse association between citrus fruit intake and oral cancer, meaning that the more citrus fruits one consumes, the less oral cancer is seen.[763] The same was found for breast and pancreatic cancers.[764,765]

In light of all these scientific findings, and the knowledge that CBD and limonene from citrus essential oils both influence GABA receptors as well as 5-HT serotonin receptors, one could understand why the combination of CBD with various essential oils from citrus fruits could be beneficial.

Note: As many citrus essential oils contains furocoumarin derivatives which are known to cause phototoxicity, be careful with the topical use of these oils. Many cases of skin damage have been described in medical literature.
[766,767,768,769,770]

It would be prudent not to use these oils topically if the skin will be exposed to the sun within the subsequent 48 to 72 hours.

Ocotea

There is a limited amount of published studies on ocotea in the medical literature. Ocotea essential oils are typically rich in camphor and safrole. One article describes the significant anti-inflammatory and gut-protecting activity of *Ocotea quixos* essential oil.[771] Another study found that ocotea essential oil possesses potent and safe antithrombotic activity attributable to its antiplatelet (prevents clumping of blood platelets) and vasorelaxant (widening of blood vessels) effects.[772]

Ocotea has also shown to be beneficial in managing diabetes and inflammation.[773] There is currently no literature or published information on ocotea and CB receptors. However, as you just saw, ocotea supports healthy blood sugar levels and so does CBD. That would make a combination of CBD and ocotea essential interesting for people with blood sugar level issues.

Ylang Ylang

The essential oil from *Cananga odorata*, also called ylang ylang, is typically used in aromatherapy as an aphrodisiac, to reduce blood pressure, and to improve cognitive function[774].

One study demonstrated that both acute and chronic ylang ylang exposure showed anxiolytic effects, like reduced stress and fear. The authors of that study believed that ylang ylang and its major constituent benzyl benzoate might act on the 5-HTnergic (activation of serotonin receptors) and DAnergic (activation of dopamine receptors) pathways.[775] Another study confirmed that activation of the serotonergic receptors in the hippocampus area of the brain by ylang ylang results in an anxiolytic effect.[776]

Ylang ylang is called a harmonizing essential oil. Aromatherapy using ylang ylang with 24 healthy volunteers resulted in a significant reduction of blood pressure and pulse rate as well as significant increase of subjective attentiveness and alertness compared to an odorless placebo.[777] A similar study using a topical application of ylang ylang essential oil also found a significant decrease of blood pressure while significantly increasing the temperature of the skin. In the same study, subjects in the ylang ylang oil group rated themselves calmer and more relaxed than subjects in the control group.[778] Another study concluded that women had improved self-esteem when using ylang ylang.[779]

Ylang ylang essential oil has a long history of use in the fragrance and food industry. To date, there has been no indication that its estimated average consumption from food flavoring use (0.0001mg/kg/day) has led to any adverse human health effects. The authors of this study concluded that at the current level of intake as a food ingredient, ylang ylang essential oil does not pose a health risk to humans.[780] The same may not be said for insects, as studies showed that ylang ylang essential oil can work against ticks.[781]

Ylang ylang essential oil contains 13 to 22% BCP[782,783] and therefore can bind to CB receptors. In addition, it has similar effects on the cardiovascular system to CBD, so a combination of both may be interesting for people with a troubled cardiovascular system. The same goes for those living in stress or fear, since both CBD and ylang ylang essential oil support a low stress life.

Cinnamon Bark

Cinnamon is one of the most important and popular spices worldwide, not just for cooking but also for traditional and modern medicine. Historically, it has mostly been used in folk medicine to treat respiratory and digestive ailments. This plant/spice has a documented use in Ayurvedic medicine for over 5000 years.

Cinnamomum verum (formerly C. *zeylanicum*) is a medicinal plant which is generally called "true cinnamon tree" or "Ceylon cinnamon tree." More than 80 compounds were identified from different parts of cinnamon, including its bark. One analysis of the essential oil showed the presence of 13 components. (E)-cinnamaldehyde was found as the major component.[784] Cinnamaldehyde and camphor have been reported to be the major components of the essential oils from cinnamon stem root bark.

Cinnamon extracts and cinnamon bark essential oil have antioxidant, antimicrobial, antidiabetic, blood pressure-lowering, cholesterol-lowering, wound healing-promoting, and liver-protecting benefits and have been successfully used in cases of Alzheimer's disease, diabetes, osteoporosis, arthritis, and arteriosclerosis.[785,786,787,788,789]

Cinnamon has also been used as an antidote for various natural and chemical toxins.[790] But the main benefits of cinnamon bark seem to be in the area of blood sugar and lipid/cholesterol regulation. Studies found that cinnamon has an insulin-mimetic effect.[791] Cinnamon can activate insulin-receptor-kinases and inhibit insulin-receptor-phosphatases, and therefore acts as an enhancer of insulin-receptor function and inhibitor of the enzyme that blocks insulin-receptor attachment.[792]

Cinnamon also contains polyphenolic compounds like rutin, catechin, quercetin, and kaempferol which all have insulin-like activity.[793] One clinic trial suggested that the higher the starting blood sugar levels are (like in poorly controlled diabetes), the better the effects of cinnamon might be.[794]

Another study found that daily cinnamon intake resulted in reduced serum glucose, triglyceride, LDL cholesterol, and total cholesterol in people with type 2 diabetes. The authors concluded that the inclusion of cinnamon will reduce risk factors associated with diabetes and cardiovascular diseases.[795]

Yet another study looking at similar endpoints demonstrated that cinnamon supplementation reduced blood sugar, HbA1c (a marker to measure the average blood sugar levels over the past two to three months), triglyceride, triglyceride to HDL ratio, and blood pressure. It also increased HDL (the "good" cholesterol) levels and eGFR (glomerular filtration rate, a measure of kidney function which often suffers over time in diabetic patients) in patients with type 2 diabetes.[796] Other studies also described that cinnamon supplementation significantly reduced blood triglycerides and total cholesterol.[797]

In summary, cinnamon has shown to have beneficial effects on diabetes and metabolic syndromes, therefore optimizing blood sugar and blood lipid levels. Like many other plants, cinnamon also contains BCP and can to bind to CB2 receptors. Cinnamon bark essential oil has up to 8% BCP.[798] Both CBD and cinnamon bark essential oil support healthy blood sugar levels.

Valerian

About 50% of the adult population in the United States experiences sleeping problems.[799] Valerian has been used for centuries as a remedy for sleep disorders.[800] Modern research shows that valerian and valerian essential oil effects are mediated through brain GABA receptors.[801,802] GABA receptor activation has shown to be beneficial in sleep disorders.[803]

A large review found that valerian improves sleep quality without producing negative side-effects.[804] Another study revealed that valerian is helpful in patients with mild to moderate insomnia, while having inconsistent effects in anxiety disorders.[805]

Some have suggested that valerian might interact with other drugs such as chemotherapy medication in cancer patients. However, a closer analysis demonstrated that there is no specific evidence questioning its safety, including in cancer patients.[806] Since both valerian and CBD influence similar receptors, they could be combined to support healthy and beneficial sleep functions.

Roman Chamomile

Chamomile is a well-known medicinal plant species and has been used in folk medicine for a long time.[807] Chamomile is mostly represented by the two common varieties German Chamomile (*Chamomilla recutita*) and Roman Chamomile (*Chamaemelum nobile*). Chamomile preparations are widely used in the cosmetic industry. It has also been used for its abdominal cramp relaxing properties.[808]

The ancient Pharmacopoeia of Württemberg (1741) described the benefits of this plant and its uses of being a carminative (substance that relieves flatulence), painkiller, diuretic, and digestive aid. In the Mediterranean region, extracts from this plant are often used after meals to prevent indigestion.

Several studies with Roman chamomile essential oil described its antibacterial and anti-inflammatory benefits.[809] It has been used for centuries for various skin, oral cavity and gums, and respiratory tract bacterial infections. Another study using an aqueous extract found a significant reduction in blood pressure as well as good diuretic (kidney supporting) effects.[810] One clinical study found that Roman chamomile also calms the skin after UV exposure, explaining why this plant has been used in skin products for such a long time.[811]

But Roman chamomile has also been used as a mild sedative to calm nerves and reduce anxiety as well as to treat hysteria, nightmares, insomnia and other sleep problems.[812] One study demonstrated the significant benefits and safety of chamomile extract in regards to

227

improving sleep quality among elderly people.[813] Inhalation of Roman chamomile essential oil has also shown to reduce depression.[814]

Another study using aromatherapy with a blend of lavender, Roman chamomile, and neroli demonstrated the anxiolytic effects of this blend in a cardiac intensive care unit. The authors concluded that aromatherapy effectively reduced the anxiety levels and increased the sleep quality of cardiac patients admitted to the ICU.[815]

Roman chamomile essential oil contains up to 10% BCP.[816] The cardiovascular effects such as increased blood flow, widening of blood vessels, and reduction of blood pressure, the skin protecting and wound healing supporting properties, as well as the calming effects are common to CBD and Roman chamomile. This opens opportunities to potentially combine these two plant compounds.

Clove

Clove is native to Indonesia but can be found in several parts of the world today. Clove deserves special attention because its antioxidant and antimicrobial activity is higher than many fruits, vegetables, and other spices.[817,818] One study found that the antioxidant free-radical scavenging activity of clove oil was superior to many other compounds.[819]

Clove extracts have long been used as an antiseptic in oral infections.[820] Researchers found that clove essential oil has a natural activity against a large number of oral pathogens.[821] It could also be used as a remedy for bad breath.[822] Interestingly, clove oil has also been used to improve depression.[823] Other neurological benefits come from the fact that clove oil can reverse both short and long-term memory deficits.[824]

Clove essential oil has significant anti-inflammatory properties.[825] It has also been shown that clove essential oil works through opioid receptors to reduce pain.[826,827] The analgesic properties of clove essential oil have been reported by various authors.[828]

Like many other plants, clove also contains BCP (up to 12%)[829] and has the ability to bind to CB2 receptors.[830] The fact that CBD and clove are involved in pain modulation and have powerful antibacterial properties creates an interesting opportunity to combine both to explore benefits in painful conditions and pathological oral or skin conditions.

Cypress

Extracts from cypress trees have long been used for relaxation, the common cold, coughs, insect repellency, and cardiovascular effects. One study showed that cypress essential oil has antimicrobial and antibiofilm properties. The authors suggested that it can therefore be used as a natural preservative ingredient in food and/or pharmaceuticals.[831]

It was also suggested that pinene (one of the main constituents in essential oils from trees) may interact with the phytocannabinoids CBD, CBN, and CBG to provide an enhanced antibacterial effect, specifically for the treatment of MRSA (a special strain of bacteria), which is often found in hospitals and is resistant to many antibiotics and other drug-resistant pathogens.[832] Overall, the antimicrobial activity of cypress essential oil has been well documented in the medical literature.[833]

The essential oil of hinoki, a cypress found in Northeast Asia, demonstrated insect-repellent activity.[834] Other studies with hinoki cypress essential oil also showed that it has therapeutic potential against respiratory inflammation-related diseases.[835] This explains why cypress has been used in folk medicine to treat the common cold and cough.[836]

Another study using aromatherapy on volunteers found that olfactory stimulation by hinoki cypress essential oil induced physiological relaxation, including benefits to the cardiovascular system.[837] The same was found when student volunteers touched hinoki wood with their naked feet.[838]

Cypress essential oil has also shown to have anti-diabetic properties and cardiovascular beneficial effects due to its ability to inhibit protein glycation and because of its high antioxidant activity.[839] Glycation of proteins (attachment of sugar molecules to some proteins) is a hallmark of advanced glycation end products (AGE) that cause premature aging of skin and internal organs.[840]

Little is known, and no literature exists to date, on the interaction of CBD and cypress extracts such as essential oils. However, the beneficial effects of both on the cardiovascular system, antiaging, and skin health make the combination of CBD and cypress essential oil an intriguing option.

Sandalwood

Sandalwood essential oil has been utilized topically for centuries in both Ayurvedic and Chinese medicine. Sandalwood (*Santalum album*) essential oil is an anti-inflammatory, antimicrobial, and anti-proliferative agent.

It has shown success in clinical trials for the treatment of acne, psoriasis, eczema, common warts, and molluscum contagiosum, which is a common and often harmless skin condition caused by a poxvirus.[841] Sandalwood oil has been called an attractive, natural therapeutic compound to treat chronic and acute inflammatory skin disorders.[842]

Natural substances like sandalwood are seeing an increase in popularity as they have shown good antimicrobial activity against difficult to treat bacteria such as MRSA.[843] It is well known that bacteria, fungi, and viruses have a reduced ability to develop resistance to botanicals.[844]

Santalol, a sesquiterpene isolated from sandalwood (up to 55% of the plant components), is known for a variety of therapeutic properties including anti-inflammatory, antioxidant, antiviral, antibacterial activities, as well as for its anti-cancer activity.

One study showed chemo-preventive and anti-cancer effects of sandalwood essential oil and α-santalol without causing toxic side-effects in a variety of tumor models including melanoma, non-melanoma, breast, prostate, and skin cancer.[845,846] Its effect on skin cancers is especially well documented.[847,848,849,850] But the anticancer effects were also impressive in bladder cancer and oral cancer.[851,852]

It is very important to know that smell receptors have been found not just on the skin but also in various organs.[853,854] One study described the wound healing benefits to the skin when sandalwood essential oil binds to these olfactory receptors called OR2AT4.[855] The same type of receptor is also involved in regulating hair growth and has been suggested as an interesting target in hair loss.[856]

Isn't it fascinating to learn that humans and animals not only benefit from essential oils scents by smelling them through the nose but also by activating smell receptors outside the smell-enabled nose?

It is also interesting to know that cancers seem to contain a reduced amount of smell receptors compared to healthy cells, which could be significant in the pathogenesis of cancers.[857] In the end, a lot may just come down to scents, whether we smell them or not, because scents might be one of the ways various cells within our body communicate. It is likely one of the reasons why essential oils can be so powerful for health, beauty, and wellness in general.

There is plenty of scientific evidence to suggest benefits from the combination of CBD with sandalwood essential oil, especially for the support of healthy skin. The combination of these two compounds could not only support healthy skin via antioxidant, anti-inflammatory, and anti-cancer effects on skin cells, but also by recreating the entourage effect around CBD by adding santalol and other botanical compounds from sandalwood essential oil to pure CBD isolates.

232

Helichrysum

Helichrysum plays an important role in the traditional medicine of Mediterranean countries. This plant, and its essential oil, have most commonly been used for the treatment of health disorders such as allergies, colds, cough, skin, liver and gallbladder disorders, inflammation, infections, and sleeplessness. [858]

In fact, it has been reported that helichrysum has phytocannabinoid properties.[859,860] To be more specific, helichrysum contains compounds from the CBD family, like cannabigerol (CBG) and cannabigerolic acid (CBGA).[861]

Research has shown that helichrysum essential oil has good antimicrobial properties.[862] Helichrysum is also known for its skin-protecting benefits such as its anti-inflammatory, anti-erythematous, and photoprotective activities.[863] The anti-inflammatory activity of *Helichrysum italicum* can be explained by multiple effects, including inflammatory enzyme inhibition and free-radical scavenging activity, both important for healthy skin.[864] The anti-inflammatory and antioxidant activities of a compound called apigenin are believed to be responsible for the wound healing benefits of helichrysum.[865]

Essential oil of *Helichrysum italicum* contains up to 5% BCP.[866] The phytocannabinoids found in helichrysum are also known to interact with some of the same receptors as CBD.[867] These facts create an interesting opportunity to combine CBD with helichrysum to explore benefits in skin health.

Black Pepper

Black pepper (*Piper nigrum*) essential oil contains about 25 to 35% β-caryophyllene (BCP), 10 to 15% limonene, about 10% pinenes, up to 4% thujene, 3% myrcene, 2% humulene, and 1% guaienes among other terpenes, oxides, ketones, aldehydes, carboxylic acids, and furanocoumarins.[868] Overall, black pepper is very rich in terpenoids with 30 to 70% monoterpenes, and 33 to 60% sesquiterpenes. As we saw earlier, β-caryophyllene binds selectively to CB2 receptors.

Studies suggested that black pepper essential oil might be a good therapeutic candidate for a variety of health conditions including wound care and metabolic diseases[869], tick infestation [870], oxidative stress[871,872], infection, inflammation, pain, and even cancer.[873] One study topically applied a pain cream made with black pepper, peppermint, lavender, and marjoram essential oils on 60 patients and found this blend to be better than a placebo cream, indicating the pain-relief activity of one or all of these essential oils.[874]

One study looked at a completely different use for black pepper essential oil, namely its topical application in problematic intravenous catheter insertions in patients with nonvisible or difficult to find veins. The essential oil was compared to standard-of-care procedures by nurses, such as application of heating pads and tactile stimulation of the veins (tapping on the skin above the veins). Topical black pepper application was clearly superior and resulted in twice the amount of visibility of veins and only half the attempts to successfully cannulate the veins.[875]

Piperine, an ingredient found in black pepper, significantly improves absorption of many compounds and inhibits phase I and phase II metabolism in the liver, resulting in higher bioavailability of natural compounds. Some studies demonstrated a multifold increase in bioavailability (up to six times) when using a new piperidine nano-formulated CBD and THC.[876,877]

Guineensine, another ingredient found in black pepper, works by inhibiting cellular uptake of the endocannabinoid anandamide. However, like piperine, guineensine is mostly lost during the distillation process. So black pepper in the form of essential oil might not be a good solution to improve the bioavailability of CBD. Nevertheless, black pepper essential oil can still be combined with CBD to take advantage of other ingredients of the essential oils such as BCP, limonene, pinenes, or others.

Sage

Sage (*Salvia officinalis*) essential oil contains up to 33% BCP. The oil can also contain up to 50% thujone (α-thujone and β-thujone combined).[878] α-thujone by itself is a GABA-A receptor antagonist that can cause convulsions and death when administered in large amounts.[879]

In fact, it was believed that thujone was the cause of absinthism after the consumption of a popular French wormwood spirit absinthe. This mental syndrome includes hallucinations, sleeplessness, and convulsions. Some authors made the connection between this drink and the famous painter Vincent van Gogh as well as artists and writers of the time like Henri de Toulouse-Lautrec and Charles Baudelaire, all known to have unstable emotions.[880]

During his last two years, van Gogh experienced fits with hallucinations that have been attributed to a congenital psychosis. But it is well known that during that time the painter was a heavy consumer of herbal spirits, including those made from wormwood.[881] The author of this article even suggested that the strange behaviors of van Gogh, such as eating paint, could have been an effort to balance terpenes chemically connected to thujone. For a while it was also speculated that van Gogh's preference for yellow colors came from the heavy consumption of absinthe.[882]

More recent studies and reviews made the authors doubt that thujone alone is the real cause for his mental problems.[883] This was confirmed by another study showing that thujone in absinthe and herbal medicines is rapid-acting and readily detoxified.[884]

However, when investigating the metabolites of α-thujone, it was found that one metabolite in particular, called 7-hydroxy-α-thujone, is less toxic than α-thujone itself. But it is present in doses seven times higher than α-thujone in the brain. Therefore, 7-hydroxy-α-thujone, together with α-thujone, could negatively affect GABA receptors leading to neurotoxicity when wormwood or sage essential oils are used in larger amounts.

Not only was thujone found to have affinity for CB1 and CB2 receptors, but sage also contains up to 33% BCP. It is certainly an interesting essential oil to combine with CBD. However, one group of scientists suggested that thujone alone was not strong enough to elicit meaningful responses on the CB receptors.[885] Therefore, sage essential oil could be added to CBD mostly to enhance the binding of BCP to CB receptors. It should also only be used in small amounts since the thujone and its metabolites can have negative effects on GABA receptors as mentioned above.

Rue or Ruta

Ruta, or "rue", is a plant of medicinal and culinary importance native to the Mediterranean region of southern Europe and northern Africa and the Balkans. The medical uses include treatment of skin diseases such as psoriasis and vitiligo, sedation, and fighting against cutaneous lymphoma. Certain components of this plant have the ability to bind directly to CB receptors.[886] The compound rutamarin showed selective affinity to the CB2 receptor.[887]

This fact makes ruta essential oils an interesting addition to blend with CBD if one intends to support stress-reduction and a healthy sleep pattern and/or reduce anxiety.

Take Away Message
- Quality matters when choosing an essential oil company.
- The information provided in this book is not intended to replace any medical advice.
- The addition of essential oils to CBD allows for a re-creation of the entourage effect.
- Both copaiba and marijuana contain significant amounts of β-caryophyllene (BCP).
- BCP selectively binds to CB2 receptors.

- CBD binds to some of the exact same receptors like lavender.
- Peppermint and CBD sometimes have the same effect and other times the opposite.
- Frankincense contains IA which binds to transient receptor potential vanillin (TRPV) receptors. CBD has also shown to bind to these receptors.
- CBD and limonene from citrus essential oils both influence GABA receptors as well as 5-HT serotonin receptors.
- Ylang ylang essential oil contains 13 to 22% BCP and therefore can bind to CB receptors. It also has similar effects on the cardiovascular system to CBD.
- Since both valerian and CBD influence similar receptors, they could be combined to support healthy and beneficial sleep functions.
- The cardiovascular effects, skin protecting and wound healing supporting properties, and calming benefits are common to both CBD and Roman chamomile.
- CBD and clove are involved in pain modulation and have powerful antibacterial properties.
- Sandalwood essential oil and CBD both support healthy skin.
- The phytocannabinoids found in helichrysum are known to interact with some of the same receptors as CBD.
- Sage essential oil could be added to CBD mostly to enhance the binding of BCP to CB receptors.
- The compound rutamarin, found in ruta essential oil, may support stress-reduction and a healthy sleep pattern and/or reduce anxiety.

Putting It All Together

So, you could recreate the entourage effect by adding essential oils or other plant compounds to CBD isolate. The beauty of this concept is that we can create a variety of blends, each containing an exact amount of CBD and essential oils, thereby accomplishing certain health-supporting effects. By changing the type and/or amount of essential oil(s), we can create different ways to support our body.

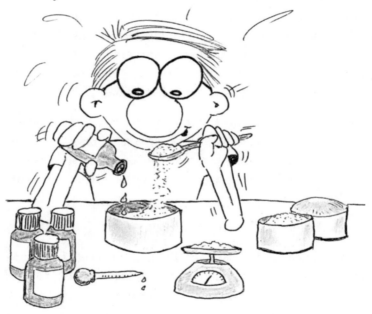

Blending CBD with Essential Oils

The listing of my combinations of CBD with essential oils is just that: a description of my personal experiences and uses of blends. Do not confuse this with a doctor's prescription to use CBD and/or essential oils for medical conditions. At this point in time, it would be illegal for me to suggest that you could use any of my personal blends to treat your medical condition(s).

In no way is this book intended as medical advice or treatment suggestions. Please always consult with your healthcare provider and physician if you have any medical conditions. Do not rely on books such as this one, or on a selection of medical articles like those listed, as the biased opinions of each author, including myself, can influence the article selection and the understanding of a reader on the subject matter. The FDA has not reviewed or approved any statements made in this book.

CBD could be combined with a variety of essential oils to create products such as lotions, creams, rubs, shampoos, hair serums, tinctures, edibles and drinkables, capsules, suppositories, and more. The possibilities are truly endless.

Formulation and Bioavailability

I mentioned earlier that orally administered CBD has extremely poor bioavailability and that certain natural substances can increase its absorption, potentially increasing its bioavailability. For example, research has shown that co-administration of dietary lipids has the potential to substantially increase the exposure to orally administered marijuana and marijuana-based medicines.[888]

One study revealed that oral co-administration of CBD with lipids can substantially increase their intestinal lymphatic transport.[889] Another study showed that piperine, curcumin, and resveratrol could enhance absorption of a CBD-based product.[890]

So, I have been trying to use a variety of food-based products to enhance absorption. As CBD is fat-soluble and mixes poorly with water, use fatty oils to dissolve the CBD isolate powder. In addition, oils such as olive, hemp, sesame, flax seed, or avocado oils also mix well with essential oils. Essential oils by themselves are also a good medium to dissolve CBD isolate powder. However, there is no scientific literature on whether essential oils improve absorption of CBD.

But how much of a blend should be created? In the beginning I experimented with 5ml and 10ml vials because I did not want to waste valuable CBD and essential oils on unsuccessful mixtures. Just to try, I mixed some CBD isolate with water and as expected, the fat-soluble CBD did not mix with water at any temperature. This is the reason why several companies are working on or already offer water-soluble CBD formulations.

Then I tried to blend CBD with an alcohol such as vodka, tequila, or rum since alcohol is a good solvent. Alcoholic CBD tinctures have also a long history of use, and interestingly, CBD-spiked cocktails are emerging as a new trend in some bars around the world. Since alcohol is amphipathic, which means that it contains polar and nonpolar ends, it can mix with water (which is polar) and also with oil (which is non-polar).

At first, it looked like it would never blend. But heating the vial under hot running water achieved a good mixing of alcohol with CBD. It also originally looked like the essential oils seemed to blend well, but after a while they always separated and started to float to the top.

The addition of curcumin only partly helped to dissolve the essential oils into the blend. In fact, curcumin, whether added as powder or liposomal formulated liquid, always settled to some extent at the bottom. A liposome is a little bubble created in the lab with at least one double-layer of fat on the outside, which facilitates the binding to fatty cell membranes. Liposomes can be used as a vehicle for administration of nutrients and pharmaceutical drugs. In fact, companies are now working on liposomal CBD formulations.

Then I started blending CBD and essential oils with olive and avocado oils. Essential oils quickly mixed with both the olive or avocado oil, but the CBD isolate powder often settled at the bottom when using olive oil. Interestingly, I did not see that with avocado oil. So nowadays, I blend the CBD isolate with avocado oil and a variety of essential oils.

I then add a few drops of liposomal curcumin, and all these compounds mix well, even at room temperature, eliminating the need to use hot running water to help with the blending. Again, this is my personal experience making mixtures that are not created in a specialized laboratory. I am sure that with the help of professional equipment I could achieve better results. But most people don't have access to a lab like that either, so these are my realistic suggestions.

My Personal Blends to Support Healthy Body Functions

I originally started with blends containing 10, 20, and then 40mg of CBD. I worked my way up until I found the dose that worked for me. I typically do not use more than one blend per day, otherwise the amount of CBD and/or essential oils would add up too quickly, increasing the risk of overdosing. Although CBD has been found to be safe up to daily doses of 6,000mg, the risk of side effects increases with higher doses.

In addition, several studies mentioned that CBD in moderate doses worked better compared to either a low or high dose, probably highlighting the fact that extremes are likely not optimal for achieving homeostasis. More is not always better.

Supporting a Restful Sleep

Like many others, I have occasional problems falling asleep, especially since I travel a lot and often cross multiple time zones. By the way, I never carry CBD with me when I travel. The uncertainty of the laws would make this too risky. In May 2019, the TSA changed their rules regarding allowing hemp and marijuana products to pass security, both in checked and carry-on luggage. However, the language used on the TSA website is so unclear that for the moment I suggest that you travel without hemp or marijuana products. And if you do, make sure that you have at least a medical prescription for it in your possession.

There have just been too many reports of travelers arrested because they had a CBD product with them. Remember, even if you can easily order CBD products to be delivered to your home, travel across state lines might still be illegal, depending on how and where the CBD was produced and which state lines you cross.

So how do I support healthy sleep? CBD combined with copaiba, lavender, cedarwood, valerian, ylang ylang, Roman chamomile, frankincense, and orange essential oils.

When blending these ingredients in a 50ml bottle, I use 10 grams of CBD isolate powder, 5ml (100 drops) copaiba essential oil, 5ml lavender essential oil (100 drops), 2ml cedarwood essential oil (40 drops), 2ml valerian essential oil (40 drops), 2ml ylang ylang essential oil (40 drops), 2ml Roman chamomile essential oil (40 drops), 2ml frankincense essential oil (40 drops), and 2ml orange essential oil (40 drops).

The remainder of the 50ml bottle is then filled with avocado oil. Finally, I add 5 drops of a liposomal curcumin into the blend and shake it well. Each milliliter of the blend then contains 250mg of CBD, which is the nightly dose I found to be just perfect for me. Remember, different people will need different amounts of CBD. I administer this dose sublingually, keep it in my mouth for about 2 minutes, and then swallow.

Supporting healthy muscles and joints

I work out most days of the week and like many others, I sometimes feel it in my joints, bones, and muscles. So, I have been blending CBD with copaiba, lavender, peppermint, clove, black pepper, and frankincense essential oils. When using CBD to support a healthy musculoskeletal system, I typically use both internal and external applications. For ingestion, I make a blend similar to the one previously mentioned (the difference is basically the essential oils used). The amount of CBD per milliliter ranges between 100 and 250mg.

Topically, I use a pain cream. I take 3 grams of a natural essential oil-based pain cream, add the aforementioned essential oils, plus wintergreen essential oil (3 drops of each), mix those with CBD isolate, and then blend with the cream. Per three grams of cream I use about 100mg of CBD isolate and about a total of 1ml of essential oils. The more I feel my bones, joints, and muscles, the more often I apply the CBD-enhanced cream, which increases the amount of CBD administered. Despite having experienced good results, I have not had the means of studying the amount of CBD absorbed through my skin.

Cardiovascular

As you read earlier in the book, cardiovascular diseases are still the leading cause of death worldwide. Since I was born with a defective heart valve and had cardiovascular issues when I was obese, I now regularly consume natural products supporting my cardiovascular health. Since CBD has the power to support a healthy cardiovascular system (heart and blood vessels) I like to blend CBD together with essential oils known to support the same. The oils I have been using for this purpose include copaiba, lavender, ylang ylang, cypress, helichrysum, Roman chamomile, rosemary, ocotea, and cinnamon bark.

For this cardiovascular blend, I use double the amount of copaiba, lavender, ylang ylang, and cypress essential oils compared to the helichrysum, Roman chamomile, rosemary, ocotea, and cinnamon bark essential oils. I typically prepare 10ml at a time which lasts for about 10 days.

For the CBD aspect of this blend, I typically use a dose of 100 to 300mg per ml. Why not more? I have a rather low blood pressure and since CBD is known to lower blood pressure, I have been a little careful with the dose. This just shows you that the use and dosage of CBD products should be personalized. So, I blend one to three grams of CBD isolate with about five to 10 drops of each of the essential oils and then use avocado oil to fill up the 10ml vial. At the end, one drop of liposomal curcumin is added.

Supporting a Healthy Brain and Healthy Nerves

To maintain a healthy central and peripheral nervous system, I use essential oils that have shown to support cognition as well as healthy brain blood flow, like copaiba, frankincense, helichrysum, sandalwood, cedarwood, peppermint, rosemary, and lemon. You could basically add each essential oil made from a spice to the blend, as most of these oils have shown to support healthy brain function.

Similar to the cardiovascular blend, I create 10ml batches and use them within 10 days. Each milliliter will contain 100 to 300mg of CBD. I frequently use only 100mg of CBD in the cardiovascular or neurological blends, because there are no good studies to date analyzing the chronic use of CBD over several years. And because I travel frequently, I often take a break from consuming CBD unless I travel to a country where I can legally obtain and consume CBD isolates.

As for the blend, I typically use one to three grams of CBD isolate in a 10ml vial. This is then mixed with 10 drops of each copaiba, frankincense, helichrysum, sandalwood, cedarwood, peppermint, rosemary, and lemon essential oils. The blend is finalized by adding one drop of liposomal curcumin and avocado oil to fill the remaining space.

Supporting a Healthy Gut

A healthy gut also means a healthy brain. When I use any of the mentioned blends with a daily CBD dose of about 50 to 300mg, I will also get benefits for my gastrointestinal system. It will also support my microbiome, which in turn is so important for brain function and my immune system.

Supporting the gut is paramount, and that is why I consume probiotics, prebiotics, as well as healthy fatty acids such as omega-3 and omega-7 fatty acids every day. Several times a week I consume hemp seeds or hemp hearts, which are full of wonderful fatty acids and proteins. I eat or drink them together with my einkorn granola or chocolate protein drinks. And once more, I would like to mention how a healthy lifestyle can support basically every organ system in the body, including the endocannabinoid system. Combine that with some CBD and essential oils and the support will be enhanced.

Supporting Healthy Skin, Healthy Beauty, and Healthy Wound Healing

The skin is not just important for looks, but also for a healthy immune system, detoxification, and even hormone production. The fact that the ECS plays a role in maintaining a healthy skin shows us that good skin is paramount for maintaining homeostasis in our body.

The ECS as well as some essential oils have shown to nicely support healthy wound healing. The fact that our skin has both smell and taste receptors that can be activated by flavors found in some essential oils led me to the concept of blending them with CBD in the form of a cream.

One of my favorite skin-supporting plants is sandalwood. This is why I use a sandalwood cream as a base to mix with CBD and additional essential oils. Similar to my muscle/joint cream, I use 100mg of CBD isolate mixed with one milliliter of essential oil (about 3 drops of each) per three grams of cream. The essential oils I use for this skin cream are copaiba, sandalwood, lavender, frankincense, cistus, helichrysum, and geranium.

As I have never found any of the white CBD isolate residual on my skin, I assume most of it is being absorbed. And because both CBD and essential oils also have strong antioxidant properties, the benefits extend from supporting healthy skin and healthy wound healing to antiaging of the skin. What could be better than feeling better and looking better at the same time?

Supporting a Healthy Immune System, Healthy Bones, and a Healthy Antioxidant Status

I originally used to create a separate blend to support my immune system. But then I realized that things were getting complicated, and that I almost had too many choices. Each of the aforementioned blends will automatically support a healthy immune system, healthy bones, and healthy eyes.

My most frequently used blend is my sleep supporting mixture. The CBD contained in that blend, benefitting from the entourage effects of the essential oils used, will most likely cover my goal when it comes to a healthy immune system, bones, and eyes. I have also noticed, that despite frequent travel in cramped spaces such as airplanes, trains, or cars, I do not get sick anymore. This is astonishing since up to 20 to 70% of airplane passengers can get flu-like symptoms within 10 days of their travel.[891,892]

Connecting the Dots

As mentioned before, the published research on combining CBD with essential oils is basically non-existent. I think, based on the current state of science, that the combination of CBD with one or more essential oils could be a good idea because they have similar properties and effects, or even bind to the same type of receptor.

However, it cannot necessarily be concluded that mixing them enhances either the effect of CBD or the effect of the essential oil. Maybe the CBD and a particular essential oil in fact compete to bind at the same receptor, and that could lead to diminished effect. But we know that CBD has only weak binding affinity to CB2 receptors, and some of the essential oils bind quite well to it.

This, combined with the knowledge that CBD most likely works through influencing the available levels of our body's own endocannabinoid anandamide, leads me to believe that the combination of CBD with essential oils is a good idea until proven otherwise by science and/or personal experience. Looking at the current body of published literature, I still think that we can recreate the entourage effect for phytocannabinoids that is lost when using CBD isolates free of any terpenes or terpenoids. This way is also safe for those at risk to be drug tested for THC.

I would like to also mention one more time that many essential oils have been classified as dietary supplements. The FDA oversees the claims that can be made with these compounds. The same would be true for CBD. However, while I am writing this book, CBD is still officially classified by the FDA as a drug. Neither CBD (with the exception of any FDA approved CBD drug) nor essential oils have been approved by the FDA to diagnose, prevent, treat, or cure any medical condition. So why would I cite all these references regarding CBD and essential oils?

While the FDA has indicated that CBD may be classified as a dietary supplement sometime in the future, the research on this miraculous compound is increasing at an accelerated speed. To date, all conclusions indicate that CBD is safe to use and that it can be used for a variety of conditions because the endocannabinoid system in our body is in charge of balancing our organ systems.

This book has not been dedicated to any specific brand of either CBD or essential oils. It should also be noted that the studies and their scientific conclusions described in this book were not done by using certain specific brands of either CBD or essential oils. In fact, many studies use only fractions or even synthetic counterparts of natural plants. I mention all of this because the word compliance has a huge importance, especially in the world of essential oil education. The CBD world is still new, and laws and regulations are being created as you read this book.

My intention is to summarize the current scientific knowledge about CBD and the possibilities of blending CBD isolate powder with certain essential oils. My goal is to give you all the necessary scientific background for you to decide if you want to start consuming CBD and/or essential oils and thereby support healthy homeostasis of your body.

I would like to emphasize again that the blends mentioned in this book have been mixed purely to support my own health and are not intended to give you precise recipes or recommendations about what you could or should do. I am simply sharing my personal experience for you to see what I have been putting together and why.

While I was researching medical literature for several years to finally write this book, I had many "Aha!" moments.

For example, years ago a very good, smart friend of mine told me that I could use essential oils even if I didn't know the exact mechanism by which it works. He mentioned that the body will know what to do with the essential oil. This was at first a complete mystery to me. How could my body just know what to do with it? My scientific brain did not process this statement very well.

But our body was created to work together with plants. Plants are not just beautiful flowers to look at or healthy foods like vegetables or fruits. They also serve us in a completely different way. Plants and humans were created to work together to achieve homeostasis in the human body. We have been gifted with an entire system intended to support our health, wellness, and beauty.

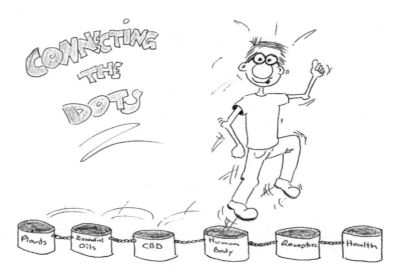

Figure 15: Connecting the dots

It is time to connect the dots. Plants and their extracts contain compounds intended to attach to some receptors in the human (and animal) body. By doing so, they either directly or indirectly help us to be in homeostasis. And when we are in homeostasis, we are healthy.

My friend was absolutely right. You don't have to know everything for something to work.

My Wish for You

First, I hope you enjoyed reading this book. Being educated about a subject gives you power. Power to know about it for yourself. Power to educate others. Power to select the correct products when it comes to CBD. Power to correctly consume CBD. Power to know which beneficial effects can be enjoyed when consuming CBD alone or in combination with essential oils. Power raises self-confidence, and self-confidence is empowering. It is a positive cycle to be in.

Second, I hope that the political and legal landscape continues to move in a direction that will empower you to legally use your newly acquired knowledge without fear. I want you to be empowered to walk into any dispensary or to look at any web site and know what you are seeing. I want you to be empowered to know what to look for when it comes to those who sell or distribute CBD and CBD-related products. I want you to be empowered to start experiencing the benefits of CBD.

Third, I want to encourage you to start experimenting with CBD in conjunction with certain plants or essential oils gained from those plants. Equipped with that knowledge you will be able to increase absorption, bioavailability, and the beneficial effects CBD can have on your body. For some of you the world of hemp and CBD is new, and for others the world of essential oils is new. And for some, this might be your first contact with either of the two.

Both worlds are fascinating, and as you gain more knowledge in either one of them, you will start to see how you and your family, your pets, and your environment will be able to benefit from these newly gained skills.

I also want you also to be aware that the medical and scientific literature does not yet contain a lot of information about the combination of CBD and essential oils. It seems that no one to date has yet bridged that gap on a scientific level. I wish I could give you more scientific proof when it comes to the combination of hemp and marijuana products with essential oils. However, this field will first have to be developed in the coming years.

I feel honored that a very good friend of mine, who left this world way too early, taught me some of his highly specialized knowledge about essential oils. This special knowledge enabled me to experiment for the past few years with the combination of CBD and essential oils. He watched me mix and blend and contributed whenever he saw an opportunity for improvement or even a chance to try something new. I am eternally grateful for that friendship.

Finally, if you have never experienced the world of essential oils and would like to be introduced to these fascinating natural treasures that God has entrusted us with, you can contact my team and me for more information. We would be happy to help you by sharing our vison, our knowledge, and our personally preferred brands of CBD and essential oils. If you wish to join me on this journey, please use the contact information provided on the next page.

Join our Team!

Never experienced CBD or essential oils?
Only want the best for your body, your
home, and your family?

Contact us at <u>cbd@doctoroli.com</u>!

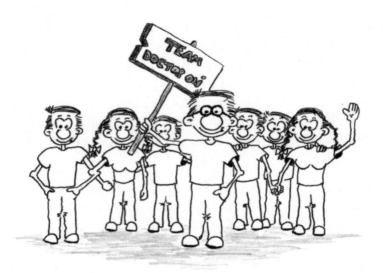

Other Resources from

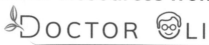

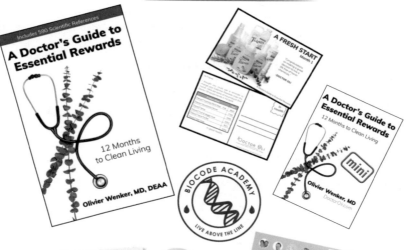

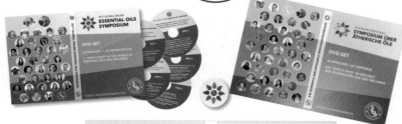

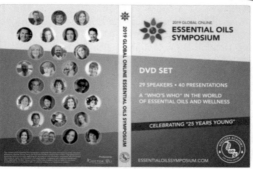

www.doctoroli.com

References:

[1] Watts G: Cannabis confusions. BMJ. 2006 Jan 21; 332(7534): 175–176. doi: 10.1136/bmj.332.7534.175. PMID: 16424501.

[2] ABC News: DNA research uncovers new cannabis strain. www.abc.net.au /news/2005-09-16/dna-research-uncovers-new-cannabis-strain/2104694.

[3] Small E. Evolution and classification of Cannabis sativa (marijuana, hemp) in relation to human utilization. Bot. Rev. 2015;81:189–294.

[4] Piomelli D, Russo EB. The Cannabis sativa Versus Cannabis indica Debate: An Interview with Ethan Russo, MD. Cannabis Cannabinoid Res. 2016;1(1):44-46. doi:10.1089/can.2015.29003.ebr.

[5] Flora of North America: Cannabis sativa. www.efloras.org /florataxon.aspx?flora_id=1&taxon_id=200006342.

[6] Pollio A: The Name of Cannabis: A Short Guide for Nonbotanists. Cannabis Cannabinoid Res. 2016; 1(1): 234–238. doi: 10.1089/can.2016.0027. PMID: 28861494.

[7] Sawler J, Stout JM, Gardner KM, Hudson D, Vidmar J, Butler L, Page JE, Myles S: The Genetic Structure of Marijuana and Hemp. PLoS One. 2015 Aug 26;10(8):e0133292. doi: 10.1371/journal.pone.0133292. PMID: 26308334.

[8] Government of the District of Columbia. Department of Health. History of Medical Cannabis. doh.dc.gov/sites/default/files/dc/sites/doh/publication /attachments/Medical%20Cannabis%20An%20Introduction %20to%20the%20Biochemistry%20and%20Pharmacology.pdf.

[9] Advanced holistic Health. 10,000-year History of Marijuana use in the World. www.advancedholistichealth.org/history.html.

[10] The antique Cannabis Book. Medical Cannabis: A Short Graphical History of Greece & Rome. antiquecannabisbook.com/chap2B/Greco_Roman/Greek-Roman.htm.

[11] Ryz NR, Remillard DJ, Russo EB. Cannabis Roots: A Traditional Therapy with Future Potential for Treating Inflammation and Pain. Cannabis Cannabinoid Res. 2017;2(1):210-216. doi:10.1089/can. 2017. 0028.

[12] Wikipedia. De Materia Medica.

[13] Ancient World Review. Cannabis In Ancient Greece: The Smoke Of The Oracles? www.ancientworldreview.com/2017/03/cannabis-in-ancient-greece-the-smoke-of-the-oracles.html.

[14] The antique Cannabis Book. Claudius Galen (130 – 200 AD). antiquecannabisbook.com/chap2B/Greco_Roman/Greek-Roman.htm.

[15] Butrica J: The Medical Use of Cannabis Among the Greeks and Romans. Journal of Cannabis Therapeutics, Vol. 2(2) 2002.

[16] Frazzetto G. Does marijuana have a future in pharmacopoeia?. EMBO Rep. 2003;4(7):651-3. doi: 10.1038/sj.embor.embor893.

[17] Massachusetts Institute of Technology MIT. The People's History. The Thistle. Volume 13, Number 2: Sept./Oct., 2000. www.mit.edu/~thistle/ v13/2/history.html.

[18] Encyclopedia Britannica: Hemp Plant. www.britannica.com/plant/hemp.

[19] World History: Hemp and Our Founding Fathers. worldhistory.us/american-history/hemp-and-our-founding-fathers. php.

[20] National Constitution Center. Busting some myths about the Founding Fathers and marijuana. Constitution Daily. constitutioncenter.org/blog/busting-some-myths-about-the-founding-fathers-and-marijuana.

[21] Nightingale P: A Brief History of Marijuana in the United States and a Case for Legalization in Pennsylvania. PCRG.org: www.pcrg.org/wp-content/uploads/2008/07/SNN-NORML-Presentation.pdf.

[22] Wikipedia. William Brooke O'Shaughnessy. en.wikipedia.org/wiki/William_Brooke_O%27Shaughnessy.

[23] Wikipedia: Pure Food and Drug Act. en.wikipedia.org/wiki/Pure_Food_and_Drug_Act.

[24] Halperin A: Marijuana: is it time to stop using a word with racist roots? The Guardian. Jan 2018. theguardian.com/society/2018/jan/29/marijuana-name-cannabis-racism

[25] Foundation for Economic Education: The Racist Roots of Marijuana Prohibition. fee.org/articles/the-racist-roots-of-marijuana-prohibition.

[26] US Legal: Marijuana Tax Act Law and Legal Definition. definitions.uslegal.com/m/marijuana-tax-act%20.

[27] Aggarwal SK, Carter GT, Sullivan MD, ZumBrunnen C, Morrill R, Mayer JD: Medicinal use of cannabis in the United States: historical perspectives, current trends, and future directions. J Opioid Manag. 2009 May-Jun;5(3):153-68. PMID: 19662925.

[28] Justicia, U.S. Supreme Court: Leary v. United States, 395 U.S. 6 (1969). supreme.justia.com/cases/federal/us/395/6.

[29] Department of Justice. Drug Enforcement Agency (DEA): Controlled Substance Schedules. www.deadiversion. usdoj.gov/schedules.

[30] The U.S. Drug Enforcement Agency DEA: Establishment of a New Drug Code for Marihuana Extract. www.federalregister.gov/documents/2016/12/14/2016-29941/establishment-of-a-new-drug-code-for-marihuana-extract.

[31] Hilderbrand RL. Hemp & Cannabidiol: What is a Medicine?. Mo Med. 2018;115(4):306-309. PMID: 30228748.

[32] The U.S. Food and Drug Administration FDA: FDA approves first drug comprised of an active ingredient derived from marijuana to treat rare, severe forms of epilepsy. www.fda.gov/newsevents/newsroom/pressannouncements/ucm611046.htm.

[33] The U.S. Drug Enforcement Agency DEA: FDA-approved drug Epidiolex placed in schedule V of Controlled Substance Act. www. dea.gov/press-releases/2018/09/27/fda-approved-drug-epidiolex-placed-schedule-v-controlled-substance-act.

[34] U.S. Food and Drug Administration. Statement from FDA Commissioner. www.fda.gov/NewsEvents/Newsroom/PressAnnouncements/ucm628988.htm? fbclid=IwAR3y5y1aWS5N6fVAq280-d4yL44ewv-F0K7y-74EqDFFuyNtrSrqiDiPlt8.

[35] Chu W, Michail N, Tay C: CBD regulation: Global clampdown or treading a careful path to acceptance? www.nutraingredients-usa.com/Article/2019/03/04/CBD-regulation-Global-clampdown-or-treading-

a-careful-path-to-acceptance?utm_source=copyright&
utm_medium=OnSite&utm_campaign=copyright.

[36] Baron EP: Comprehensive Review of Medicinal Marijuana, Cannabinoids, and Therapeutic Implications in Medicine and Headache: What a Long Strange Trip It's Been .... Headache. 2015 Jun;55(6):885-916. doi: 10.1111/head.12570.

[37] Matador Network: No, CBD is not legal in all 50 States. matadornetwork.com/read/cbd-laws-united-states.

[38] Green Roads: Is CBD Legal in 2019? The Legal Status Of CBD In 50 States. www.greenroadsworld.com/pages/is-cbd-legal.

[39] Hemp Basics: General Hemp Information, Uses, Facts. www.hempbasics.com/shop/general-hemp-information.

[40] Yonavjak L: Industrial Hemp: A Win-Win For The Economy And The Environment. Forbes Online: www.forbes.com/sites/ashoka/ 2013/05/29/industrial-hemp-a-win-win-for-the-economy-and-the-environment/#3b3d93b289b1.

[41] Yang Y, Lewis MM, Bello AM, Wasilewski E, Clarke HA, Kotra LP: Cannabis sativa (Hemp) Seeds, Δ9-Tetrahydrocannabinol, and Potential Overdose. Cannabis Cannabinoid Res. 2017 Oct 1;2(1):274-281. doi: 10.1089/can.2017.0040. PMID: 29098190.

[42] U.S. National Library of Medicine. Amino acids. medlineplus.gov/ ency/article/002222.htm.

[43] Alvares TS, Conte CA, Paschoalin VM, Silva JT, Meirelles Cde M, Bhambhani YN, Gomes PS: Acute l-arginine supplementation increases muscle blood volume but not strength performance. Appl Physiol Nutr Metab. 2012 Feb;37(1):115-26. doi: 10.1139/h11-144.

[44] Bode-Böger SM, Böger RH, Galland A, Tsikas D, Frölich JC: L-arginine-induced vasodilation in healthy humans: pharmacokinetic–pharmacodynamic relationship. Br J Clin Pharmacol. 1998 Nov; 46(5): 489–497. doi: 10.1046/j.1365-2125.1998.00803.x.

[45] Vasdev S, Gill V: The antihypertensive effect of arginine. Int J Angiol. 2008 Spring; 17(1): 7–22. PMID: 22477366.

[46] Pahlavani N, Jafari M, Sadeghi O, Rezaei M, Rasad H, Rahdar HA, Entezari MH: L-arginine supplementation and risk factors of cardiovascular diseases in healthy men: a double-blind randomized clinical trial. F1000Res. 2017;3:306. doi:10.12688/f1000research.5877.2.

[47] Young SN: L-Tyrosine to alleviate the effects of stress? J Psychiatry Neurosci. 2007 May; 32(3): 224. PMID: 17476368.

[48] Callaway JC: Hempseed as a nutritional resource: An overview. Euphytica (2004) 140: 65. Doi: 10.1007/s10681-004-4811-6.

[49] Luo Q, Yan X, Bobrovskaya L, Ji M, Yuan H, Lou H, Fan P: Anti-neuroinflammatory effects of grossamide from hemp seed via suppression of TLR-4-mediated NF-κB signaling pathways in lipopolysaccharide-stimulated BV2 microglial cells. Mol Cell Biochem. 2017 Apr;428(1-2):129-137. doi: 10.1007/s11010-016-2923-7.

[50] The U.S. Food And Drug Administration FDA. FDA Statement: Statement from FDA Commissioner Scott Gottlieb, M.D., on signing of the Agriculture Improvement Act and the agency's regulation of products containing

cannabis and cannabis-derived compounds. www.fda.gov/
NewsEvents/Newsroom/PressAnnouncements/ucm628988.htm.
[51] Merriam-Webster Dictionary: Definition of dioecious. www.merriam-webster.com/dictionary/dioecious.
[52] Merriam-Webster Dictionary: Definition of dioecious. www.merriam-webster.com/dictionary/ monoecious.
[53] Huchelmann A, Boutry M, Hachez C. Plant Glandular Trichomes: Natural Cell Factories of High Biotechnological Interest. Plant Physiol. 2017;175(1):6-22. doi: 10.1104/pp.17.00727.
[54] Dhifi W, Bellili S, Jazi S, Bahloul N, Mnif W: Essential Oils' Chemical Characterization and Investigation of Some Biological Activities: A Critical Review. Medicines (Basel). 2016;3(4):25. doi:10.3390/medicines3040025.
[55] Gilbert AN, DiVerdi JA: Consumer perceptions of strain differences in Cannabis aroma. PLoS One. 2018;13(2):e0192247. doi:10.1371/journal.pone.0192247.
[56] Substance Abuse Center for Behavioral Health Statistics and Quality. Results from the 2015 National Survey on Drug Use and Health: Detailed Tables. SAMHSA. www.samhsa.gov/data/sites/default/files/NSDUH-DetTabs-2015/NSDUH-DetTabs-2015/NSDUH-DetTabs-2015.pdf.
[57] Bridgeman MB, Abazia DT. Medicinal Cannabis: History, Pharmacology, And Implications for the Acute Care Setting. P T. 2017;42(3):180-188. PMID: 28250701.
[58] Turner AR, Agrawal S: StatPerls; Marijuana Toxicity. 2018. www.ncbi.nlm.nih.gov/books/NBK430823.
[59] Eaton DK, Kann L, Kinchen S, Shanklin S, Ross J, Hawkins J, Harris WA, Lowry R, McManus T, Chyen D, Lim C, Whittle L, Brener ND, Wechsler H; Centers for Disease Control and Prevention (CDC): Youth risk behavior surveillance - United States, 2009. MMWR Surveill Summ. 2010 Jun 4;59(5):1-142. PMID: 20520591.
[60] Pizzorno J. What Should We Tell Our Patients About Marijuana (Cannabis indica and Cannabis sativa)?. Integr Med (Encinitas). 2016;15(6):8-12. PMID: 28223891.
[61] Gallop. One in eight U.S. adults say they smoke marijuana. www.gallop.com/poll/194195/.
[62] van Nuijs AL, Castiglioni S, Tarcomnicu I, Postigo C, Lopez de Alda M, Neels H, Zuccato E, Barcelo D, Covaci A: Illicit drug consumption estimations derived from wastewater analysis: a critical review. Sci Total Environ. 2011 Sep 1;409(19):3564-77. doi: 10.1016/j.scitotenv.2010.05.030.
[63] Thomas KV, Bijlsma L, Castiglioni S, Covaci A, Emke E, Grabic R, et al.: Comparing illicit drug use in 19 European cities through sewage analysis. Sci Total Environ. 2012 Aug 15;432:432-9. doi: 10.1016/j.scitotenv.2012.06.069.
[64] Steinmetz K: 420 Day: Why There Are So Many Different Names for Weed. Time: time.com/4747501/420-day-weed-marijuana-pot-slang.
[65] Wikipedia: Etymology of cannabis. en.wikipedia.org/wiki/Etymology_of_cannabis.
[66] Russo E: History of Cannabis and Its Preparations in Saga, Science, and Sobriquet. Chemistry & Biodiversity. 2007 Nov. 4(8):1614-48. doi:10.1002/cbdv.200790144.

[67] Civilized: Why is Weed called Weed? www.civilized. life/articles/why-is-weed-called-weed.

[68] Dictionary.com: Why is Marijuana also called pot? www.dictionary.com/e/pot-marijuana.

[69] Borgelt LM, Franson KL, Nussbaum AM, Wang GS: The pharmacologic and clinical effects of medical cannabis. Pharmacotherapy. 2013 Feb;33(2):195-209. doi: 10.1002/phar.1187.

[70] Schrot RJ, Hubbard JR: Cannabinoids: Medical implications. Ann Med. 2016;48(3):128-41. doi: 10.3109/07853890.2016.1145794.

[71] Kramer JL: Medical marijuana for cancer. CA Cancer J Clin. 2015 Mar;65(2):109-22. doi: 10.3322/caac.21260.

[72] Parmar JR, Forrest BD, Freeman RA: Medical marijuana patient counseling points for health care professionals based on trends in the medical uses, efficacy, and adverse effects of cannabis-based pharmaceutical drugs. Res Social Adm Pharm. 2016 Jul-Aug;12(4):638-54. doi: 10.1016/j.sapharm.2015.09.002.

[73] Kim PS, Fishman MA: Cannabis for Pain and Headaches: Primer. Curr Pain Headache Rep. 2017 Apr;21(4):19. doi:10.1007/s11916-017-0619-7.

[74] Baron EP: Comprehensive Review of Medicinal Marijuana, Cannabinoids, and Therapeutic Implications in Medicine and Headache: What a Long Strange Trip It's Been. Headache. 2015 Jun;55(6):885-916. doi: 10.1111/head.12570.

[75] Clark P, Dubensky J, Evans A, Bhatt H, Ayala A, Umapathy S: The Ethics of Medical Marijuana: Government Restrictions vs. Medical Necessity (An Update). The Internet Journal of Law, Healthcare, and Ethics IJLHE 2019. ispub.com/IJLHE.

[76] Grotenhermen F: Pharmacokinetics and pharmacodynamics of cannabinoids. Clin Pharmacokinet. 2003;42(4):327-60. doi: 10.2165/00003088-200342040-00003.

[77] Freeman D, Dunn G, Murray RM, et al: How cannabis causes paranoia: using the intravenous administration of Ω9-tetrahydrocannabinol (THC) to identify key cognitive mechanisms leading to paranoia. Schizophr Bull. 2014;41(2):391-9. doi: 10.1093/schbul/sbu098.

[78] Li MC, Brady JE, DiMaggio CJ, Lusardi AR, Tzong KY, Li G: Marijuana use and motor vehicle crashes. Epidemiol Rev. 2012;34:65-72. doi: 10.1093/epirev/mxr017.

[79] Asbridge M, Hayden JA, Cartwright JL: Acute cannabis consumption and motor vehicle collision risk: systematic review of observational studies and meta-analysis. BMJ. 2012 Feb 9;344:e536. doi: 10.1136/bmj.e536.

[80] Bédard M, Dubois S, Weaver B: The impact of cannabis on driving. Can J Public Health. 2007 Jan-Feb;98(1):6-11. PMID: 17278669.

[81] Janowsky DS, Meacham MP, Blaine JD, Schoor M, Bozzetti LP: Marijuana effects on simulated flying ability. Am J Psychiatry. 1976 Apr;133(4):384-8. doi: 10.1176/ajp.133.4.384.

[82] Leirer VO, Yesavage JA, Morrow DG: Marijuana carry-over effects on aircraft pilot performance. Send toAviat Space Environ Med. 1991 Mar; 62(3):221-7. PMID: 1849400.

[83] Vaidya JG, Block RI, O'Leary DS, Ponto LB, Ghoneim MM, Bechara A: Effects of chronic marijuana use on brain activity during monetary decision-making. Neuropsychopharmacology. 2012 Feb;37(3):618-29. doi: 10.1038/npp.2011.227.

[84] Bolla KI, Eldreth DA, Matochik JA, Cadet JL: Neural substrates of faulty decision-making in abstinent marijuana users. Neuroimage. 2005 Jun;26(2):480-92. doi: 10.1016/j.neuroimage.2005.02.012.

[85] Ashton H: Adverse effects of cannabis. Adverse Drug Reaction Bulletin: October 2002 - Volume - Issue 216 - p 827–830.

[86] The National Institute on Drug Abuse: What are marijuana's long-term effects on the brain? www.drugabuse.gov/publications/research-reports/marijuana/what-are-marijuanas-long-term-effects-brain.

[87] Batalla A, Bhattacharyya S, Yücel M, Fusar-Poli P, Crippa JA, Nogué S, Torrens M, Pujol J, Farré M, Martin-Santos R.: Structural and functional imaging studies in chronic cannabis users: a systematic review of adolescent and adult findings. PLoS One. 2013;8(2):e55821. doi: 10.1371/journal.pone.0055821.

[88] Prestifilippo JP, Fernández-Solari J, de la Cal C, Iribarne M, Suburo AM, Rettori V, McCann SM, Elverdin JC: Inhibition of salivary secretion by activation of cannabinoid receptors. Exp Biol Med (Maywood). 2006 Sep;231(8):1421-9. PMID: 16946411.

[89] Fernandez-Solari J, Prestifilippo JP, Vissio P, Ehrhart-Bornstein M, Bornstein SR, Rettori V, Elverdin JC: Anandamide injected into the lateral ventricle of the brain inhibits submandibular salivary secretion by attenuating parasympathetic neurotransmission. Braz J Med Biol Res. 2009 Jun;42(6):537-44. PMID: 19448903.

[90] Agrawal A, Lynskey MT: The genetic epidemiology of cannabis use, abuse and dependence. Addiction. 2006 Jun;101(6):801-12. doi: 10.1111/j.1360-0443.2006.01399.x

[91] Olthuis JV, Darredeau C, Barrett SP: Substance use initiation: the role of simultaneous polysubstance use. Drug Alcohol Rev. 2013 Jan;32(1):67-71. doi: 10.1111/j.1465-3362.2012.00470.x.

[92] Sartor CE, Agrawal A, Lynskey MT, Duncan AE, Grant JD, Nelson EC, Madden PA, Heath AC, Bucholz KK: Cannabis or alcohol first? Differences by ethnicity and in risk for rapid progression to cannabis-related problems in women. Psychol Med. 2013 Apr;43(4):813-23. doi: 10.1017/S0033291712001493.

[93] Barrett SP, Darredeau C, Pihl RO: Patterns of simultaneous polysubstance use in drug using university students. Hum Psychopharmacol. 2006 Jun;21(4):255-63. doi: 10.1002/hup.766.

[94] Secades-Villa R, Garcia-Rodríguez O, Jin CJ, Wang S, Blanco C. Probability and predictors of the cannabis gateway effect: a national study. Int J Drug Policy. 2014;26(2):135-42. doi: 10.1016/j.drugpo.2014.07.011.

[95] The National Institute on Drug Abuse: Is marijuana a gateway drug? www.drugabuse.gov/publications/research-reports/marijuana/marijuana-gateway-drug.

[96] Stolberg SG: Government Study Of Marijuana Sees Medical Benefits. The New York Times. 2018.www.nytimes.com/1999/03/18/us/government-study-of-marijuana-sees-medical-benefits.html.

[97] van Ours JC: Is cannabis a stepping-stone for cocaine? J Health Econ. 2003 Jul;22(4):539-54. doi: 10.1016/S0167-6296(03)00005-5

[98] Centers for disease Control and Prevention Understanding the Epidemic. Record Overdose Deaths. www.cdc.gov/drugoverdose/epidemic/index.html.

[99] Sidney S, Beck JE, Tekawa IS, Quesenberry CP, Friedman GD. Marijuana use and mortality. Am J Public Health. 1997;87(4):585-90. PMID: 9146436.

[100] Fischer B, Imtiaz S, Rudzinski K, Rehm J. Crude estimates of cannabis-attributable mortality and morbidity in Canada-implications for public health focused intervention priorities. J Public Health (Oxf). 2015;38(1):183-8. doi: 10.1093/pubmed/fdv005.

[101] Harris R: NPR Public Health. (2018). Opioid Use Lower In States That Eased Marijuana Laws. www.npr.org/sections/health-shots/2018/04/02/598787768/opioid-use-lower-in-states-that-eased-marijuana-laws.

[102] Bradford AC, Bradford WD, Abraham A, Bagwell Adams G: Association Between US State Medical Cannabis Laws and Opioid Prescribing in the Medicare Part D Population. JAMA Intern Med. 2018;178(5):667–672. doi:10.1001/jamainternmed.2018.0266.

[103] Grinspoon P: Cannabidiol (CBD) -what we know and what we don't. Harvard Medical School Health Blog. www.health.harvard.edu/blog/cannabidiol-cbd-what-we-know-and-what-we-dont-2018082414476.

[104] Thomas A, Baillie GL, Phillips AM, Razdan RK, Ross RA, Pertwee RG: Cannabidiol displays unexpectedly high potency as an antagonist of CB1 and CB2 receptor agonists in vitro. Br J Pharmacol. 2007 Mar; 150(5):613-23. doi: 10.1038/sj.bjp.0707133.

[105] Pertwee RG: The diverse CB1 and CB2 receptor pharmacology of three plant cannabinoids: delta9-tetrahydrocannabinol, cannabidiol and delta9-tetrahydrocannabivarin. Br J Pharmacol. 2008 Jan;153(2):199-215. doi: 10.1038/sj.bjp.0707442.

[106] Niesink RJ, van Laar MW. Does Cannabidiol Protect Against Adverse Psychological Effects of THC?. Front Psychiatry. 2013;4:130. doi:10.3389/fpsyt.2013.00130.

[107] Englund A, et al: Cannabidiol inhibits THC-elicited paranoid symptoms and hippocampal-dependent memory impairment. J Psychopharmacol. 2013 Jan;27(1):19-27.doi:10.1177/0269881112460109.

[108] Wright MJ Jr, Vandewater SA, Taffe MA: Cannabidiol attenuates deficits of visuospatial associative memory induced by $\Delta(9)$ tetrahydrocannabinol. Br J Pharmacol. 2013 Dec;170(7):1365-73. doi: 10.1111/bph.12199.

[109] Boggs DL, Nguyen JD, Morgenson D, Taffe MA, Ranganathan M: Clinical and Preclinical Evidence for Functional Interactions of Cannabidiol and $\Delta9$-Tetrahydrocannabinol. Neuropsychopharmacology. 2018 Jan;43(1):142-154. doi: 10.1038/npp.2017.209.

[110] Todd SM, Zhou C, Clarke DJ, Chohan TW, Bahceci D, Arnold JC: Interactions between cannabidiol and $\Delta9$-THC following acute and repeated dosing:

Rebound hyperactivity, sensorimotor gating and epigenetic and neuroadaptive changes in the mesolimbic pathway. Eur Neuropsychopharmacol. 2017 Feb;27(2):132-145. doi: 10.1016/j.euroneuro.2016.12.004.

[111] Merrick J, Lane B, Sebree T, et al. Identification of psychoactive degradants of cannabidiol in simulated gastric and physiological fluid. Cannabis Cannabinoid Res. 2016;1:102–112. doi: 10.1089/can.2015.0004.

[112] Nahler G, Grotenhermen F, Zuardi AW, Crippa JAS: A Conversion of Oral Cannabidiol to Delta9-Tetrahydrocannabinol Seems Not to Occur in Humans. Cannabis Cannabinoid Res. 2017;2(1):81–86. doi:10.1089/can.2017.0009.

[113] Bergamaschi MM, Queiroz RH, Zuardi AW, Crippa JA: Safety and side effects of cannabidiol, a Cannabis sativa constituent. Curr Drug Saf. 2011 Sep 1;6(4):237-49. PMID: 22129319.

[114] Hampson AJ, Grimaldi M, Axelrod J, Wink D. Cannabidiol and (-)Delta9-tetrahydrocannabinol are neuroprotective antioxidants. Proc Natl Acad Sci U S A. 1998;95(14):8268–8273.

[115] McPartland JM, Duncan M, Di Marzo V, Pertwee RG. Are cannabidiol and $\Delta(9)$ -tetrahydrocannabivarin negative modulators of the endocannabinoid system? A systematic review. Br J Pharmacol. 2015;172(3):737–753. doi:10.1111/bph.12944.

[116] Schwilke EW, Schwope DM, Karschner EL, et al. Delta9-tetrahydrocannabinol (THC), 11-hydroxy-THC, and 11-nor-9-carboxy-THC plasma pharmacokinetics during and after continuous high-dose oral THC. Clin Chem. 2009;55(12):2180–2189. doi:10.1373/clinchem.2008. 122119.

[117] Lemberger L, Crabtree RE, Rowe HM: 11-hydroxy- 9 - tetrahydrocannabinol: pharmacology, disposition, and metabolism of a major metabolite of marihuana in man. Science. 1972 Jul 7;177(4043):62-4. PMID: 5041775.

[118] Sharma P, Murthy P, Bharath MM. Chemistry, metabolism, and toxicology of cannabis: clinical implications. Iran J Psychiatry. 2012;7(4):149–156. PMID: 23408483.

[119] Volkow ND, Baler RD, Compton WM, Weiss SR. Adverse health effects of marijuana use. N Engl J Med. 2014;370(23):2219–2227. doi:10.1056/NEJMra1402309.

[120] Webb CW, Webb SM. Therapeutic benefits of cannabis: a patient survey. Hawaii J Med Public Health. 2014;73(4):109–111.

[121] Grant I, Atkinson JH, Gouaux B, Wilsey B. Medical marijuana: clearing away the smoke. Open Neurol J. 2012;6:18–25. doi:10.2174/1874205X01206010018.

[122] Bar-Lev Schleider L, Mechoulam R, Lederman V, Hilou M, Lencovsky O, Betzalel O, Shbiro L, Novack V: Prospective analysis of safety and efficacy of medical cannabis in large unselected population of patients with cancer. Eur J Intern Med. 2018 Mar;49:37-43. doi: 10.1016/j.ejim.2018.01.023.

[123] Lim K, See YM, Lee J. A Systematic Review of the Effectiveness of Medical Cannabis for Psychiatric, Movement and Neurodegenerative Disorders. Clin Psychopharmacol Neurosci. 2017;15(4):301–312. doi:10.9758/cpn.2017.15.4.301.

[124] Bornheim LM, Grillo MP: Characterization of cytochrome P450 3A inactivation by cannabidiol: possible involvement of cannabidiol-hydroxyquinone as a P450 inactivator. Chem Res Toxicol. 1998 Oct;11(10):1209-16. doi: 10.1021/tx9800598.

[125] Marcu JP, et al: Cannabidiol enhances the inhibitory effects of delta9-tetrahydrocannabinol on human glioblastoma cell proliferation and survival. Mol Cancer Ther. 2010 Jan;9(1):180-9. doi: 10.1158/1535-7163.MCT-09-0407.

[126] Russo E, Guy GW: A tale of two cannabinoids: the therapeutic rationale for combining tetrahydrocannabinol and cannabidiol. Med Hypotheses. 2006;66(2):234-46. doi: 10.1016/j.mehy.2005.08.026.

[127] Khan, B. A., Warner, P., Wang, H. (2014). Antibacterial properties of hemp and other natural fibre plants: A review. Bio Res. 9(2),3642-3659.

[128] Andre CM, Hausman JF, Guerriero G: Front. Plant Sci., 04 February 2016. doi.org/10.3389/fpls.2016.0001.

[129] Appendino G, Gibbons S, Giana A, Pagani A, Grassi G, Stavri M, Smith E, Rahman MM: Antibacterial Cannabinoids from Cannabis sativa: A Structure–Activity Study. J. Nat. Prod., 2008, 71 (8), pp 1427–1430 doi: 10.1021/np8002673.

[130] Hao XM, Yang Y, An LX, Wang, JM, Han L: Study on antibacterial mechanism of hemp fiber. Adv. Mat. Res. (2014). 887–888, 610–613. doi: 10.4028/www.scientific.net/AMR.887-888.610.

[131] Martyny JW, Serrano KA, Schaeffer JW, Van Dyke MV: Potential exposures associated with indoor marijuana growing operations. J Occup Environ Hyg. 2013;10(11):622-39. doi: 10.1080/15459624.2013.831986.

[132] Thomas BF, Pollard GT: Preparation and Distribution of Cannabis and Cannabis-Derived Dosage Formulations for Investigational and Therapeutic Use in the United States. Front Pharmacol. 2016;7:285. doi:10.3389/fphar.2016.00285.

[133] StoneD: Cannabis, pesticides and conflicting laws: the dilemma for legalized States and implications for public health. Regul Toxicol Pharmacol. 2014 Aug;69(3):284-8. doi: 10.1016/j.yrtph.2014.05.015.

[134] Subritzky T, Pettigrew S, Lenton S: Into the void: Regulating pesticide use in Colorado's commercial cannabis markets. Int J Drug Policy. 2017 Apr;42:86-96. doi: 10.1016/j.drugpo.2017.01.014.

[135] Pizzorno J. What Should We Tell Our Patients About Marijuana (Cannabis indica and Cannabis sativa)? Integr Med (Encinitas). 2016;15(6):8-12. PMID: 28223891.

[136] Busse F, Omidi L, Timper K, Leichtle A, Windgassen M, Kluge E, Stumvoll M: Lead poisoning due to adulterated marijuana. N Engl J Med. 2008 Apr 10;358(15):1641-2. doi: 10.1056/NEJMc0707784.

[137] Russo EB: Current Therapeutic Cannabis Controversies and Clinical Trial Design Issues. Front Pharmacol. 2016;7:309. doi:10.3389/fphar.2016.00309.

[138] Raber JC, Elzinga S, Kaplan C: Understanding dabs: contamination concerns of cannabis concentrates and cannabinoid transfer during the act of dabbing. J Toxicol Sci. 2015 Dec;40(6):797-803. doi: 10.2131/jts.40.797.

[139] Sullivan N, Elzinga S, Raber JC: Determination of pesticide residues in cannabis smoke. J Toxicol.2013;2013:378168.doi:10.1155/2013/378168.

[140] Russo E. B: Pesticide contamination of cannabis in the legal market, 26th Annual Conference on the Cannabinoids, International Cannabinoid Research Society (Bukovina:), 66.

[141] Wikipedia: Supercritical carbon dioxide. en.wikipedia.org/wiki/Supercritical_carbon_dioxide

[142] Marijuana Break: The Complete Guide to CBD Extractions (CO2 Cannabis Extraction, Olive Oil and Solvents). www.marijuanabreak.com/cbd-cannabis-extraction

[143] BigSkyBotanicals: How is CBD Oil Made: A Beginners Guide to Hemp Extraction. bigskybotanicals.com/education/how-is-cbd-oil-made.

[144] Romano L, Hazekamp A: Cannabis oil: Chemical evaluation of an upcoming cannabis based medicine. Cannabinoids. 2013;1(1):1–11.

[145] Casiraghi A, Roda G, Casagni E, Cristina C, Musazzi UM, Franzè S, Rocco P, Giuliani C, Fico G, Minghetti P, Gambaro V: Extraction Method and Analysis of Cannabinoids in Cannabis Olive Oil Preparations. Planta Med. 2018 Mar;84(4):242-249. doi: 10.1055/s-0043-123074.

[146] Hazekamp A: Evaluating the Effects of Gamma-Irradiation for Decontamination of Medicinal Cannabis. Front Pharmacol. 2016 Apr 27;7:108. doi: 10.3389/fphar.2016.00108.

[147] Gertsch J, Leonti M, Raduner S, Racz I, Chen JZ, Xie XQ, Altmann KH, Karsak M, Zimmer A: Beta-caryophyllene is a dietary cannabinoid. Proc Natl Acad Sci U S A. 2008 Jul 1;105(26):9099-104. doi: 10.1073/pnas.0803601105.

[148] Raber JC, Elzinga S, Kaplan C: Understanding dabs: contamination concerns of cannabis concentrates and cannabinoid transfer during the act of dabbing. J Toxicol Sci. 2015 Dec;40(6):797-803. doi: 10.2131/jts.40.797.

[149] Malfitano AM, Basu S, Maresz K, Bifulco M, Dittel BN: What we know and do not know about the cannabinoid receptor 2 (CB2). Semin Immunol. 2014 Oct;26(5):369-79. doi: 10.1016/j.smim.2014.04.002.

[150] Di Marzo V: 'Endocannabinoids' and other fatty acid derivatives with cannabimimetic properties: biochemistry and possible physiopathological relevance. Biochim Biophys Acta. 1998 Jun 15;1392(2-3):153-75. PMID: 9630590.

[151] Wong BS, Camilleri M, Eckert D, Carlson P, Ryks M, Burton D, Zinsmeister AR: Randomized pharmacodynamic and pharmacogenetic trial of dronabinol effects on colon transit in irritable bowel syndrome-diarrhea. Neurogastroenterol Motil. 2012 Apr;24(4):358-e169. doi: 10.1111/j.1365-2982.2011.01874.x.

[152] Russo EB: Clinical Endocannabinoid Deficiency Reconsidered: Current Research Supports the Theory in Migraine, Fibromyalgia, Irritable Bowel, and Other Treatment-Resistant Syndromes. Cannabis Cannabinoid Res. 2016;1(1):154-165. Published 2016 Jul 1. doi:10.1089/can.2016.0009.

[153] Sarchielli P, Pini LA, Coppola F, Rossi C, Baldi A, Mancini ML, Calabresi P: Endocannabinoids in chronic migraine: CSF findings suggest a system failure. Neuropsychopharmacology. 2007 Jun;32(6):1384-90. doi: 10.1038/sj.npp.1301246.

[154] Giuffrida A, Leweke FM, Gerth CW, Schreiber D, Koethe D, Faulhaber J, Klosterkötter J, Piomelli D: Cerebrospinal anandamide levels are elevated in

acute schizophrenia and are inversely correlated with psychotic symptoms. Neuropsychopharmacology. 2004 Nov;29(11):2108-14. doi: 10.1038/sj.npp.1300558.

[155] Pisani V, Moschella V, Bari M, Fezza F, Galati S, Bernardi G, Stanzione P, Pisani A, Maccarrone M: Dynamic changes of anandamide in the cerebrospinal fluid of Parkinson's disease patients. Mov Disord. 2010 May 15;25(7):920-4. doi: 10.1002/mds.23014.

[156] Allen KL, Waldvogel HJ, Glass M, Faull RL: Cannabinoid (CB(1)), GABA(A) and GABA(B) receptor subunit changes in the globus pallidus in Huntington's disease. J Chem Neuroanat. 2009 Jul;37(4):266-81. doi: 10.1016/j.jchemneu.2009.02.001.

[157] Choukèr A, Kaufmann I, Kreth S, Hauer D, Feuerecker M, Thieme D, Vogeser M, Thiel M, Schelling G: Motion sickness, stress and the endocannabinoid system. PLoS One. 2010 May 21;5(5):e10752. doi: 10.1371/journal.pone.0010752.

[158] Gérard N, Pieters G, Goffin K, Bormans G, Van Laere K: Brain type 1 cannabinoid receptor availability in patients with anorexia and bulimia nervosa. Biol Psychiatry. 2011 Oct 15;70(8):777-84. doi: 10.1016/j.biopsych.2011.05.010.

[159] Engeli S: Dysregulation of the endocannabinoid system in obesity. J Neuroendocrinol. 2008 May;20 Suppl 1:110-5. doi: 10.1111/j.1365-2826.2008.01683.x.

[160] Russo EB: Clinical endocannabinoid deficiency (CECD): can this concept explain therapeutic benefits of cannabis in migraine, fibromyalgia, irritable bowel syndrome and other treatment-resistant conditions? Neuro Endocrinol Lett. 2004 Feb-Apr;25(1-2):31-9. PMID: 15159679.

[161] Maroon J, Bost J. Review of the neurological benefits of phytocannabinoids. Surg Neurol Int. 2018;9:91. Published 2018 Apr 26. doi:10.4103/sni.sni_45_18.

[162] Mechoulam R, Hanus L.: A historical overview of chemical research on cannabinoids. Chem Phys Lipids. 2000 Nov;108(1-2):1-13. PMID: 11106779.

[163] Pertwee RG. Cannabinoid pharmacology: the first 66 years. Br J Pharmacol. 2006;147 Suppl 1(Suppl 1):S163-71. doi: 10.1038/sj.bjp.0706406.

[164] Wollner HJ, Matchett JR, Levine J, Loewe S: Isolation of a Physiologically Active Tetrahydrocannabinol from Cannabis Sativa Resin. J. Am. Chem. Soc., 1942, 64 (1), pp 26–29. doi: 10.1021/ja01253a008.

[165] Mechoulam R, Shvo Y: Hashish. I. The structure of cannabidiol. Tetrahedron. 1963 Dec;19(12):2073-8. PMID: 5879214.

[166] Matsuda LA, Lolait SJ, Brownstein MJ, Young AC, Bonner TI: Structure of a cannabinoid receptor and functional expression of the cloned cDNA. Nature. 1990 Aug 9;346(6284):561-4. doi: 10.1038/346561a0.

[167] Zuardi AW: Cannabidiol: from an inactive cannabinoid to a drug with wide spectrum of action. Braz J Psychiatry. 2008 Sep;30(3):271-80. PMID: 18833429.

[168] Pertwee RG: Pharmacology of cannabinoid CB1 and CB2 receptors. Pharmacol Ther. 1997;74(2):129-80. PMID: 9336020.

[169] Nature Education: G-protein-coupled receptors (GPCRs). www.nature.com/scitable/topicpage/gpcr-14047471.

[170] Glass M, Dragunow M, Faull RL: Cannabinoid receptors in the human brain: a detailed anatomical and quantitative autoradiographic study in the fetal, neonatal and adult human brain. Neuroscience. 1997 Mar;77(2):299-318. PMID: 9472392.

[171] Galiègue S, Mary S, Marchand J, Dussossoy D, Carrière D, Carayon P, Bouaboula M, Shire D, Le Fur G, Casellas P: Expression of central and peripheral cannabinoid receptors in human immune tissues and leukocyte subpopulations. Eur J Biochem. 1995 Aug 15;232(1):54-61. PMID: 7556170.

[172] Bouaboula M, Rinaldi M, Carayon P, Carillon C, Delpech B, Shire D, Le Fur G, Casellas P: Cannabinoid-receptor expression in human leukocytes. Eur J Biochem. 1993 May 15;214(1):173-80. PMID: 8508790.

[173] Núñez E, Benito C, Pazos MR, Barbachano A, Fajardo O, González S, Tolón RM, Romero J: Cannabinoid CB2 receptors are expressed by perivascular microglial cells in the human brain: an immunohistochemical study. Synapse. 2004 Sep 15;53(4):208-13. doi: 10.1002/syn.20050.

[174] Jane E. Lauckner, Jill B. Jensen, Huei-Ying Chen, Hui-Chen Lu, Bertil Hille, Ken Mackie: GPR55 is a cannabinoid receptor that increases intracellular calcium and inhibits M current. Proceedings of the National Academy of Sciences 2008, 105 (7) 2699-2704; doi: 10.1073/pnas.0711278105.

[175] Moriconi A, Cerbara I, Maccarone M, Topai A: GPR55: Current knowledge and future perspectives of a purported "Type-3" cannabinoid receptor. Curr Med Chem. 2010;17(14):1411-29. PMID: 20166924.

[176] Yang H, Zhou J, Lehmann C: GPR55 - a putative "type 3" cannabinoid receptor in inflammation. J Basic Clin Physiol Pharmacol. 2016 May 1;27(3):297-302. doi: 10.1515/jbcpp-2015-0080.

[177] Ryberg E, Larsson N, Sjögren S, et al. The orphan receptor GPR55 is a novel cannabinoid receptor. Br J Pharmacol. 2007;152(7):1092-101. doi: 10.1038/sj.bjp.0707460.

[178] Nevalainen T, Irving AJ: GPR55, a lysophosphatidylinositol receptor with cannabinoid sensitivity? Curr Top Med Chem. 2010;10(8):799-813. PMID: 20370712.

[179] Yin H, Chu A, Li W, et al: Lipid G protein-coupled receptor ligand identification using beta-arrestin PathHunter assay. J Biol Chem. 2009;284(18):12328-38. doi: 10.1074/jbc.M806516200.

[180] Wikipedia. GPR55: en.wikipedia.org/wiki/GPR55.

[181] Whyte LS, Ryberg E, Sims NA, Ridge SA, Mackie K, Greasley PJ, Ross RA, Rogers MJ: The putative cannabinoid receptor GPR55 affects osteoclast function in vitro and bone mass in vivo. Proc Natl Acad Sci U S A. 2009 Sep 22;106(38):16511-6. doi: 10.1073/pnas.0902743106.

[182] Bab I, Ofek O, Tam J, Rehnelt J, Zimmer A: Endocannabinoids and the regulation of bone metabolism. J Neuroendocrinol. 2008 May;20 Suppl 1:69-74. doi: 10.1111/j.1365-2826.2008.01675.x.

[183] Idris AI, Ralston SH: Cannabinoids and bone: friend or foe? Calcif Tissue Int. 2010 Oct;87(4):285-97. doi: 10.1007/s00223-010-9378-8.

[184] Tam J, Trembovler V, Di Marzo V, Petrosino S, Leo G, Alexandrovich A, Regev E, Casap N, Shteyer A, Ledent C, Karsak M, Zimmer A, Mechoulam R, Yirmiya R, Shohami E, Bab I: The cannabinoid CB1 receptor regulates bone

formation by modulating adrenergic signaling. FASEB J. 2008 Jan;22(1):285-94. doi: 10.1096/fj.06-7957com.

[185] Idris AI, Ralston SH: Role of cannabinoids in the regulation of bone remodeling. Front Endocrinol (Lausanne). 2012;3:136. doi:10.3389/fendo.2012.00136 .

[186] Wikipedia: G protein-coupled receptor. en.wikipedia.org/wiki/G_protein-coupled_receptor.

[187] Weiss N: The N-Type Voltage-Gated Calcium Channel: When a Neuron Reads a Map. J Neuroscience 2008, 28 (22) 5621-5622; doi 10.1523/JNEUROSCI.1538-08.2008.

[188] Maccarrone M, Bab I, Bíró T, Cabral GA, Dey SK, Di Marzo V, Konje JC, Kunos G, Mechoulam R, Pacher P, Sharkey KA, Zimmer A: Endocannabinoid signaling at the periphery: 50 years after THC. Trends Pharmacol Sci. 2015 May;36(5):277-96. doi: 10.1016/j.tips.2015.02.008.

[189] Cancer Centers of America: What's the Difference? B-cells and T-cells. www.cancercenter.com/discussions/blog/whats-the-difference-b-cells-and-t-cells.

[190] Cano RLE, Lopera HDE: Autoimmunity: From Bench to Bedside, Introduction to T and B lymphocytes. El Rosario University Press; 2013 Jul 18. Chapter 5. www.ncbi.nlm.nih.gov/books/NBK459471.

[191] Jan TR, Su ST, Wu HY, Liao MH: Suppressive effects of cannabidiol on antigen-specific antibody production and functional activity of splenocytes in ovalbumin-sensitized BALB/c mice. Int Immunopharmacol. 2007 Jun;7(6):773-80. doi: 10.1016/j.intimp.2007.01.015.

[192] Kaplan BL, Springs AE, Kaminski NE: The profile of immune modulation by cannabidiol (CBD) involves deregulation of nuclear factor of activated T cells (NFAT). Biochem Pharmacol. 2008;76(6):726-37. doi: 10.1016/j.bcp.2008.06.022.

[193] Cabral GA, Griffin-Thomas L: Emerging role of the cannabinoid receptor CB2 in immune regulation: therapeutic prospects for neuroinflammation. Expert Rev Mol Med. 2009 Jan 20;11:e3. doi: 10.1017/S1462399409000957.

[194] Basu S, Dittel BN: Unraveling the complexities of cannabinoid receptor 2 (CB2) immune regulation in health and disease. Immunol Res. 2011 Oct;51(1):26-38. doi: 10.1007/s12026-011-8210-5.

[195] Basavarajappa BS. Neuropharmacology of the endocannabinoid signaling system-molecular mechanisms, biological actions and synaptic plasticity. Curr Neuropharmacol. 2007;5(2):81-97. PMID: 18084639.

[196] Wikipedia: Cannabinoid. en.wikipedia.org/wiki/Cannabinoid.

[197] Malfitano AM, Basu S, Maresz K, Bifulco M, Dittel BN: What we know and do not know about the cannabinoid receptor 2 (CB2). Semin Immunol. 2014;26(5):369-79. doi: 10.1016/j.smim.2014.04.002.

[198] Devane WA, Hanus L, Breuer A, Pertwee RG, Stevenson LA, Griffin G, Gibson D, Mandelbaum A, Etinger A, Mechoulam R: Isolation and structure of a brain constituent that binds to the cannabinoid receptor. Science. 1992 Dec 18;258(5090):1946-9. PMID: 1470919.

[199] Mechoulam R, Ben-Shabat S, Hanus L, Ligumsky M, Kaminski NE, Schatz AR, Gopher A, Almog S, Martin BR, Compton DR, et al: Identification of an endogenous 2-monoglyceride, present in canine gut, that binds to

cannabinoid receptors. Biochem Pharmacol. 1995 Jun 29;50(1):83-90. PMID: 7605349.

[200] UCI News. 'Love hormone' helps produce 'bliss molecules' to boost pleasure of social interactions. news.uci.edu/2015/10/26/love-hormone-helps-produce-bliss-molecules-to-boost-pleasure-of-social-interactions.

[201] Di Marzo V, De Petrocellis L: Why do cannabinoid receptors have more than one endogenous ligand? Philos Trans R Soc Lond B Biol Sci. 2012 Dec 5;367(1607):3216-28. doi: 10.1098/rstb.2011.0382.

[202] Manseau MW, Goff DC. Cannabinoids and Schizophrenia: Risks and Therapeutic Potential. Neurotherapeutics. 2015;12(4):816–824. doi:10.1007/s13311-015-0382-6.

[203] Giuffrida A, Leweke FM, Gerth CW, Schreiber D, Koethe D, Faulhaber J, Klosterkötter J, Piomelli D: Cerebrospinal anandamide levels are elevated in acute schizophrenia and are inversely correlated with psychotic symptoms. Neuropsychopharmacology. 2004 Nov;29(11):2108-14. doi: 10.1038/sj.npp.1300558.

[204] Deutsch DG. A Personal Retrospective: Elevating Anandamide (AEA) by Targeting Fatty Acid Amide Hydrolase (FAAH) and the Fatty Acid Binding Proteins (FABPs). Front Pharmacol. 2016;7:370. doi:10.3389/fphar.2016.00370.

[205] Bisogno T, Hanus L, De Petrocellis L, Tchilibon S, Ponde DE, Brandi I, Moriello AS, Davis JB, Mechoulam R, Di Marzo V: Molecular targets for cannabidiol and its synthetic analogues: effect on vanilloid VR1 receptors and on the cellular uptake and enzymatic hydrolysis of anandamide. Br J Pharmacol. 2001 Oct;134(4):845-52. doi: 10.1038/sj.bjp.0704327.

[206] Elmes MW, Kaczocha M, Berger WT, Leung K, Ralph BP, Wang L, Sweeney JM, Miyauchi JT, Tsirka SE, Ojima I, Deutsch DG: Fatty acid-binding proteins (FABPs) are intracellular carriers for Δ9-tetrahydrocannabinol (THC) and cannabidiol (CBD). J Biol Chem. 2015 Apr 3;290(14):8711-21. doi: 10.1074/jbc.M114.618447.

[207] van der Stelt M, Veldhuis WB, van Haaften GW, Fezza F, Bisogno T, Bar PR, Veldink GA, Vliegenthart JF, Di Marzo V, Nicolay K: Exogenous anandamide protects rat brain against acute neuronal injury in vivo. J Neurosci. 2001 Nov 15;21(22):8765-71. PMID: 11698588.

[208] Martín Giménez VM, Noriega SE, Kassuha DE, Fuentes LB, Manucha W: Anandamide and endocannabinoid system: an attractive therapeutic approach for cardiovascular disease. Ther Adv Cardiovasc Dis. 2018 Jul;12(7):177-190. doi: 10.1177/1753944718773690.

[209] De Petrocellis L, Melck D, Palmisano A, Bisogno T, Laezza C, Bifulco M, Di Marzo V: The endogenous cannabinoid anandamide inhibits human breast cancer cell proliferation. Proc Natl Acad Sci U S A. 1998 Jul 7;95(14):8375-80. PMID: 9653194.

[210] Schwarz H, Blanco FJ, Lotz M: Anadamide, an endogenous cannabinoid receptor agonist inhibits lymphocyte proliferation and induces apoptosis. J Neuroimmunol. 1994 Nov;55(1):107-15. PMID: 7962480.

[211] Chiurchiù V, Rapino C, Talamonti E, Leuti A, Lanuti M, Gueniche A, Jourdain R, Breton L, Maccarrone M: Anandamide Suppresses Proinflammatory T Cell Responses In Vitro through Type-1 Cannabinoid Receptor-Mediated mTOR

Inhibition in Human Keratinocytes. J Immunol. 2016 Nov 1;197(9):3545-3553. doi: 10.4049/jimmunol.1500546.

[212] Sharkey KA, Wiley JW. The Role of the Endocannabinoid System in the Brain-Gut Axis. Gastroenterology. 2016;151(2):252–266. doi:10.1053/j.gastro.2016.04.015.

[213] DiPatrizio NV. Endocannabinoids in the Gut. Cannabis Cannabinoid Res. 2016;1(1):67–77. doi:10.1089/can.2016.0001.

[214] Khasabova IA, Khasabov SG, Harding-Rose C, Coicou LG, Seybold BA, Lindberg AE, Steevens CD, Simone DA, Seybold VS: A decrease in anandamide signaling contributes to the maintenance of cutaneous mechanical hyperalgesia in a model of bone cancer pain. J Neurosci. 2008 Oct 29;28(44):11141-52. doi: 10.1523/JNEUROSCI.2847-08.2008.

[215] Schmid PC, Paria BC, Krebsbach RJ, Schmid HH, Dey SK. Changes in anandamide levels in mouse uterus are associated with uterine receptivity for embryo implantation. Proc Natl Acad Sci U S A. 1997;94(8): 4188–4192. PMID: 9108127.

[216] Pertwee RG, Fernando SR, Nash JE, Coutts AA: Further evidence for the presence of cannabinoid CB1 receptors in guinea-pig small intestine. Br J Pharmacol. 1996 Aug;118(8):2199-205. PMID: 8864562.

[217] Di Marzo V, Piscitelli F: Gut feelings about the endocannabinoid system. Neurogastroenterol Motil. 2011 May;23(5):391-8. doi: 10.1111/j.1365-2982.2011.01689.x.

[218] Ofek O, Karsak M, Leclerc N, Fogel M, Frenkel B, Wright K, Tam J, Attar-Namdar M, Kram V, Shohami E, Mechoulam R, Zimmer A, Bab I: Peripheral cannabinoid receptor, CB2, regulates bone mass. Proc Natl Acad Sci U S A. 2006 Jan 17;103(3):696-701. doi: 10.1073/pnas.0504187103.

[219] Chen J, Matias I, Dinh T, Lu T, Venezia S, Nieves A, Woodward DF, Di Marzo V: Finding of endocannabinoids in human eye tissues: implications for glaucoma. Biochem Biophys Res Commun. 2005 May 20;330(4):1062-7. doi: 10.1016/j.bbrc.2005.03.095.

[220] Sugiura T, Kishimoto S, Oka S, Gokoh M: Biochemistry, pharmacology and physiology of 2-arachidonoylglycerol, an endogenous cannabinoid receptor ligand. Prog Lipid Res. 2006 Sep;45(5):405-46. doi: 10.1016/j.plipres.2006.03.003.

[221] Flores A, Maldonado R, Berrendero F: Cannabinoid-hypocretin cross-talk in the central nervous system: what we know so far. Front Neurosci. 2013 Dec 20;7:256. doi: 10.3389/fnins.2013.00256.

[222] Cristino L, Busetto G, Imperatore R, Ferrandino I, Palomba L, Silvestri C, Petrosino S, Orlando P, Bentivoglio M, Mackie K, Di Marzo V: Obesity-driven synaptic remodeling affects endocannabinoid control of orexinergic neurons. Proc Natl Acad Sci U S A. 2013 Jun 11;110(24): E2229-38. doi: 10.1073/pnas.1219485110.

[223] Manduca A, Morena M, Campolongo P, Servadio M, Palmery M, Trabace L, Hill MN, Vanderschuren LJ, Cuomo V, Trezza V: Distinct roles of the endocannabinoids anandamide and 2-arachidonoylglycerol in social behavior and emotionality at different developmental ages in rats. Eur Neuropsychopharmacol. 2015 Aug;25(8):1362-74. doi: 10.1016/j.euroneuro.2015.04.005.

[224] Degn M, Lambertsen KL, Petersen G, Meldgaard M, Artmann A, Clausen BH, Hansen SH, Finsen B, Hansen HS, Lund TM: Changes in brain levels of N-acylethanolamines and 2-arachidonoylglycerol in focal cerebral ischemia in mice. J Neurochem. 2007 Dec;103(5):1907-16. doi: 10.1111/j.1471-4159.2007.04892.x.

[225] Di Marzo V, Hill MP, Bisogno T, Crossman AR, Brotchie JM: Enhanced levels of endogenous cannabinoids in the globus pallidus are associated with a reduction in movement in an animal model of Parkinson's disease. FASEB J. 2000 Jul;14(10):1432-8. PMID: 10877836.

[226] Baker D, Pryce G, Croxford JL, Brown P, Pertwee RG, Makriyannis A, Khanolkar A, Layward L, Fezza F, Bisogno T, Di Marzo V: Endocannabinoids control spasticity in a multiple sclerosis model. FASEB J. 2001 Feb;15(2):300-2. doi: 10.1096/fj.00-0399fje.

[227] Brose SA, Golovko SA, Golovko MY. Brain 2-Arachidonoylglycerol Levels Are Dramatically and Rapidly Increased Under Acute Ischemia-Injury Which Is Prevented by Microwave Irradiation. Lipids. 2016;51(4):487–495. doi:10.1007/s11745-016-4144-y.

[228] Stella N, Schweitzer P, Piomelli D: A second endogenous cannabinoid that modulates long-term potentiation. Nature. 1997 Aug 21;388(6644): 773-8. doi: 10.1038/42015.

[229] Rea K, Roche M, Finn DP: Supraspinal modulation of pain by cannabinoids: the role of GABA and glutamate. Br J Pharmacol. 2007 Nov;152(5):633-48. doi: 10.1038/sj.bjp.0707440.

[230] Blankman JL, Simon GM, Cravatt BF: A comprehensive profile of brain enzymes that hydrolyze the endocannabinoid 2-arachidonoylglycerol. Chem Biol. 2007 Dec;14(12):1347-56. doi: 10.1016/j.chembiol. 2007.11.006.

[231] Wenzel JM, Cheer JF: Endocannabinoid-dependent modulation of phasic dopamine signaling encodes external and internal reward-predictive cues. Front Psychiatry. 2014 Sep 1;5:118. doi: 10.3389/fpsyt.2014.00118.

[232] Morales P, Reggio PH, Jagerovic N. An Overview on Medicinal Chemistry of Synthetic and Natural Derivatives of Cannabidiol. Front Pharmacol. 2017;8:422. doi:10.3389/fphar.2017.00422.

[233] Bisogno T, Hanus L, De Petrocellis L, et al. Molecular targets for cannabidiol and its synthetic analogues: effect on vanilloid VR1 receptors and on the cellular uptake and enzymatic hydrolysis of anandamide. Br J Pharmacol. 2001;134(4):845–852. doi:10.1038/sj.bjp.0704327.

[234] Nagarkatti P, Pandey R, Rieder SA, Hegde VL, Nagarkatti M. Cannabinoids as novel anti-inflammatory drugs. Future Med Chem. 2009;1(7):1333–1349. doi:10.4155/fmc.09.93.

[235] Elmes MW, Kaczocha M, Berger WT, et al. Fatty acid-binding proteins (FABPs) are intracellular carriers for Δ9-tetrahydrocannabinol (THC) and cannabidiol (CBD). J Biol Chem. 2015;290(14):8711–8721. doi:10.1074/jbc.M114.618447.

[236] McPartland JM, Duncan M, Di Marzo V, Pertwee RG: Are cannabidiol and Δ(9)-tetrahydrocannabivarin negative modulators of the endocannabinoid system? A systematic review. Br J Pharmacol. 2015 Feb;172(3):737-53. doi: 10.1111/bph.12944.

[237] Thomas A, Baillie GL, Phillips AM, Razdan RK, Ross RA, Pertwee RG: Cannabidiol displays unexpectedly high potency as an antagonist of CB1 and CB2 receptor agonists in vitro. Br J Pharmacol. 2007 Mar;150(5): 613-23. doi: 10.1038/sj.bjp.0707133.

[238] Rollinger JM, Schuster D, Danzl B, et al. In silico target fishing for rationalized ligand discovery exemplified on constituents of Ruta graveolens. Planta Med. 2008;75(3):195-204. doi: 10.1055/s-0028-1088397.

[239] Yin H, Chu A, Li W, et al. Lipid G protein-coupled receptor ligand identification using beta-arrestin PathHunter assay. J Biol Chem. 2009;284(18):12328-38. doi: 10.1074/jbc.M806516200.

[240] Vardakou I, Pistos C, Spiliopoulou CH: Spice drugs as a new trend: Mode of action, identification and legislation. Toxicology Letters. Volume 197, Issue 3, 1 September 2010, Pages 157-162. doi.org/10.1016/j.toxlet.2010.06.002.

[241] Basavarajappa BS, Subbanna S. Potential Mechanisms Underlying the Deleterious Effects of Synthetic Cannabinoids Found in Spice/K2 Products. Brain Sci. 2019;9(1):14. doi:10.3390/brainsci9010014.

[242] Trecki J, Gerona RR, Schwartz MD: Synthetic Cannabinoid-Related Illnesses and Deaths. N Engl J Med. 2015 Jul 9;373(2):103-7. doi: 10.1056/NEJMp1505328.

[243] Adamowicz P, Meissner E, Maślanka M: Fatal intoxication with new synthetic cannabinoids AMB-FUBINACA and EMB-FUBINACA. Clin Toxicol (Phila). 2019 Feb 26:1-6. doi: 10.1080/15563650.2019.1580371.

[244] Katz KD, Leonetti AL, Bailey BC, et al. Case Series of Synthetic Cannabinoid Intoxication from One Toxicology Center. West J Emerg Med. 2016;17(3):290–294. doi:10.5811/westjem.2016.2.29519.

[245] Sweeney B, Talebi S, Toro D, Gonzalez K, Menoscal JP, Shaw R, Hassen GW: Hyperthermia and severe rhabdomyolysis from synthetic cannabinoids. Am J Emerg Med. 2016 Jan;34(1):121.e1-2. doi: 10.1016/j.ajem.2015.05.052.

[246] Durand D, Delgado LL, de la Parra-Pellot DM, Nichols-Vinueza D: Psychosis and severe rhabdomyolysis associated with synthetic cannabinoid use: A case report. Clin Schizophr Relat Psychoses. 2015 Jan;8(4):205-8. doi: 10.3371/CSRP.DUDE.031513.

[247] Varlet V. Drug Vaping: From the Dangers of Misuse to New Therapeutic Devices. Toxics. 2016;4(4):29. doi:10.3390/toxics4040029.

[248] Besli GE, Ikiz MA, Yildirim S, Saltik S: Synthetic Cannabinoid Abuse in Adolescents: A Case Series. J Emerg Med. 2015 Nov;49(5):644-50. doi: 10.1016/j.jemermed.2015.06.053.

[249] Okamoto Y, Morishita J, Tsuboi K, Tonai T, Ueda N: Molecular characterization of a phospholipase D generating anandamide and its congeners. J Biol Chem. 2004 Feb 13;279(7):5298-305. doi: 10.1074/jbc.M306642200.

[250] Murataeva N, Straiker A, Mackie K. Parsing the players: 2-arachidonoylglycerol synthesis and degradation in the CNS. Br J Pharmacol. 2014;171(6):1379–1391. doi:10.1111/bph.12411.

[251] Thors L, Alajakku K, Fowler CJ: The 'specific' tyrosine kinase inhibitor genistein inhibits the enzymic hydrolysis of anandamide: implications for anandamide uptake. Br J Pharmacol. 2007 Apr;150(7):951-60. doi: 10.1038/sj.bjp.0707172.

[252] Thors L, Belghiti M, Fowler CJ: Inhibition of fatty acid amide hydrolase by kaempferol and related naturally occurring flavonoids. Br J Pharmacol. 2008 Sep;155(2):244-52. doi: 10.1038/bjp.2008.237.

[253] Petrosino S, Di Marzo V: FAAH and MAGL inhibitors: therapeutic opportunities from regulating endocannabinoid levels. Curr Opin Investig Drugs. 2010 Jan;11(1):51-62. PMID: 20047159.

[254] Di Pasquale E, Chahinian H, Sanchez P, Fantini J. The insertion and transport of anandamide in synthetic lipid membranes are both cholesterol-dependent. PLoS One. 2009;4(3):e4989. doi: 10.1371/journal.pone.0004989.

[255] Stanley CP, O'Sullivan SE. Cyclooxygenase metabolism mediates vasorelaxation to 2-arachidonoylglycerol (2-AG) in human mesenteric arteries. Pharmacol Res. 2014;81(100):74–82. doi:10.1016/j.phrs.2014.02.001.

[256] Fowler CJ: Transport of endocannabinoids across the plasma membrane and within the cell. FEBS J. 2013 May;280(9):1895-904. doi: 10.1111/febs.12212.

[257] Quistad GB, Nomura DK, Sparks SE, Segall Y, Casida JE: Cannabinoid CB1 receptor as a target for chlorpyrifos oxon and other organophosphorus pesticides. Toxicol Lett. 2002 Sep 5;135(1-2):89-93. PMID: 12243867.

[258] Segall Y, Quistad GB, Sparks SE, Nomura DK, Casida JE: Toxicological and structural features of organophosphorus and organosulfur cannabinoid CB1 receptor ligands. Toxicol Sci. 2003 Nov;76(1):131-7. doi: 10.1093/toxsci/kfg216.

[259] Lafourcade M, Larrieu T, Mato S, Duffaud A, Sepers M, Matias I, De Smedt-Peyrusse V, Labrousse VF, Bretillon L, Matute C, Rodríguez-Puertas R, Layé S, Manzoni OJ: Nutritional omega-3 deficiency abolishes endocannabinoid-mediated neuronal functions. Nat Neurosci. 2011 Mar;14(3):345-50. doi: 10.1038/nn.2736.

[260] Khan MZ, He L: The role of polyunsaturated fatty acids and GPR40 receptor in brain. Neuropharmacology. 2017 Feb;113(Pt B):639-651. doi: 10.1016/j.neuropharm.2015.05.013.

[261] Riediger ND, Othman RA, Suh M, Moghadasian MH: A systemic review of the roles of n-3 fatty acids in health and disease. J Am Diet Assoc. 2009 Apr;109(4):668-79. doi: 10.1016/j.jada.2008.12.022.

[262] Simopoulos AP: The importance of the ratio of omega-6/omega-3 essential fatty acids. Biomed Pharmacother. 2002 Oct;56(8):365-79. PMID: 12442909.

[263] Simopoulos AP: Evolutionary aspects of diet, the omega-6/omega-3 ratio and genetic variation: nutritional implications for chronic diseases. Biomed Pharmacother. 2006 Nov;60(9):502-7. doi: 10.1016/j.biopha.2006.07.080.

[264] Simopoulos AP. An Increase in the Omega-6/Omega-3 Fatty Acid Ratio Increases the Risk for Obesity. Nutrients. 2016;8(3):128. doi:10.3390/nu8030128.

[265] Alvheim AR, Malde MK, Osei-Hyiaman D, Lin YH, Pawlosky RJ, Madsen L, Kristiansen K, Frøyland L, Hibbeln JR: Dietary linoleic acid elevates endogenous 2-AG and anandamide and induces obesity. Obesity (Silver Spring). 2012 Oct;20(10):1984-94. doi: 10.1038/oby.2012.38.

[266] Hutchins-Wiese HL, Li Y, Hannon K, Watkins BA: Hind limb suspension and long-chain omega-3 PUFA increase mRNA endocannabinoid system

levels in skeletal muscle. J Nutr Biochem. 2012 Aug;23(8):986-93. doi: 10.1016/j.jnutbio.2011.05.005.

[267] Piscitelli F, Carta G, Bisogno T, Murru E, Cordeddu L, Berge K, Tandy S, Cohn JS, Griinari M, Banni S, Di Marzo V: Effect of dietary krill oil supplementation on the endocannabinoidome of metabolically relevant tissues from high-fat-fed mice. Nutr Metab (Lond). 2011 Jul 13;8(1):51. doi: 10.1186/1743-7075-8-51.

[268] Lafourcade M, Larrieu T, Mato S, Duffaud A, Sepers M, Matias I, De Smedt-Peyrusse V, Labrousse VF, Bretillon L, Matute C, Rodríguez-Puertas R, Layé S, Manzoni OJ: Nutritional omega-3 deficiency abolishes endocannabinoid-mediated neuronal functions. Nat Neurosci. 2011 Mar;14(3):345-50. doi: 10.1038/nn.2736.

[269] McDougle DR, Watson JE, Abdeen AA, Adili R, Caputo MP, Krapf JE, Johnson RW, Kilian KA, Holinstat M, Das A: Anti-inflammatory ω-3 endocannabinoid epoxides. Proceedings of the National Academy of Sciences Jul 2017, 114 (30) E6034-E6043; doi: 10.1073/pnas.1610325114.

[270] Rodriguez-Leyva D, Pierce GN. The cardiac and haemostatic effects of dietary hempseed. Nutr Metab (Lond). 2010;7:32. doi:10.1186/1743-7075-7-32.

[271] Gavel NT, Edel AL, Bassett CM, Weber AM, Merchant M, Rodriguez-Leyva D, Pierce GN: The effect of dietary hempseed on atherogenesis and contractile function in aortae from hypercholesterolemic rabbits. Acta Physiol Hung. 2011 Sep;98(3):273-83. doi: 10.1556/APhysiol.98.2011.3.4.

[272] Prociuk MA, Edel AL, Richard MN, Gavel NT, Ander BP, Dupasquier CM, Pierce GN: Cholesterol-induced stimulation of platelet aggregation is prevented by a hempseed-enriched diet. Can J Physiol Pharmacol. 2008 Apr;86(4):153-9. doi: 10.1139/Y08-011.

[273] James JS: Marijuana and chocolate. AIDS Treat News. 1996 Oct 18;(No 257):3-4. PMID: 11363932.

[274] di Tomaso E, Beltramo M, Piomelli D: Brain cannabinoids in chocolate. Nature. 1996 Aug 22;382(6593):677-8. doi: 10.1038/382677a0.

[275] Thors L, Burston JJ, Alter BJ, et al. Biochanin A, a naturally occurring inhibitor of fatty acid amide hydrolase. Br J Pharmacol. 2010;160(3):549–560. doi:10.1111/j.1476-5381.2010.00716.x.

[276] Korte G, Dreiseitel A, Schreier P, Oehme A, Locher S, Geiger S, Heilmann J, Sand PG: Tea catechins' affinity for human cannabinoid receptors. Phytomedicine. 2010 Jan;17(1):19-22. doi: 10.1016/j.phymed.2009.10.001.

[277] Rossi S, De Chiara V, Musella A, Mataluni G, Sacchetti L, Siracusano A, Bernardi G, Usiello A, Centonze D: Caffeine drinking potentiates cannabinoid transmission in the striatum: interaction with stress effects. Neuropharmacology. 2009 Mar;56(3):590-7. doi: 10.1016/j.neuropharm.2008.10.013.

[278] Leonti M, Casu L, Raduner S, Cottiglia F, Floris C, Altmann KH, Gertsch J: Falcarinol is a covalent cannabinoid CB1 receptor antagonist and induces pro-allergic effects in skin. Biochem Pharmacol. 2010 Jun 15;79(12):1815-26. doi: 10.1016/j.bcp.2010.02.015.

[279] Leonti M, Casu L, Raduner S, Cottiglia F, Floris C, Altmann KH, Gertsch J: Falcarinol is a covalent cannabinoid CB1 receptor antagonist and induces

pro-allergic effects in skin. Biochem Pharmacol. 2010 Jun 15;79(12):1815-26. doi: 10.1016/j.bcp.2010.02.015.

[280] Purup S, Larsen E, Christensen LP. Differential effects of falcarinol and related aliphatic C(17)-polyacetylenes on intestinal cell proliferation. J Agric Food Chem. 2009;57(18):8290-6. doi: 10.1021/jf901503a.

[281] Zaini RG, Brandt K, Clench MR, Le Maitre CL: Effects of bioactive compounds from carrots (Daucus carota L.), polyacetylenes, beta-carotene and lutein on human lymphoid leukaemia cells. Anticancer Agents Med Chem. 2012 Jul;12(6):640-52. PMID: 22263789.

[282] Metzger BT, Barnes DM, Reed JD: Purple carrot (Daucus carota L.) polyacetylenes decrease lipopolysaccharide-induced expression of inflammatory proteins in macrophage and endothelial cells. J Agric Food Chem. 2008 May 28;56(10):3554-60. doi: 10.1021/jf073494t.

[283] Ligresti A, Villano R, Allarà M, Ujváry I, Di Marzo V: Kavalactones and the endocannabinoid system: the plant-derived yangonin is a novel CB1 receptor ligand. Pharmacol Res. 2012 Aug;66(2):163-9. doi: 10.1016/j.phrs.2012.04.003.

[284] Ligresti A, Villano R, Allarà M, Ujváry I, Di Marzo V: Kavalactones and the endocannabinoid system: the plant-derived yangonin is a novel CB1 receptor ligand. Pharmacol Res. 2012 Aug;66(2):163-9. doi: 10.1016/j.phrs.2012.04.003.

[285] Hassanzadeh P, Hassanzadeh A: The CB1 receptor-mediated endocannabinoid signaling and NGF: the novel targets of curcumin. Neurochem Res. 2012 May;37(5):1112-20. doi: 10.1007/s11064-012-0716-2.

[286] Quezada SM, Cross RK: Cannabis and Turmeric as Complementary Treatments for IBD and Other Digestive Diseases. Curr Gastroenterol Rep. 2019 Jan 11;21(2):2. doi: 10.1007/s11894-019-0670-0.

[287] Cherniakov I, Izgelov D, Domb AJ, Hoffman A: The effect of Pro NanoLipospheres (PNL) formulation containing natural absorption enhancers on the oral bioavailability of delta-9-tetrahydrocannabinol (THC) and cannabidiol (CBD) in a rat model. Eur J Pharm Sci. 2017 Nov 15;109:21-30. doi: 10.1016/j.ejps.2017.07.003.

[288] Bruni N, Della Pepa C, Oliaro-Bosso S, Pessione E, Gastaldi D, Dosio F. Cannabinoid Delivery Systems for Pain and Inflammation Treatment. Molecules. 2018;23(10):2478. doi:10.3390/molecules23102478.

[289] Hewlings SJ, Kalman DS. Curcumin: A Review of Its' Effects on Human Health. Foods. 2017;6(10):92. Published 2017 Oct 22. doi:10.3390/foods6100092.

[290] Olson R: Absinthe and γ-aminobutyric acid receptors. Proceedings of the National Academy of Sciences Apr 2000, 97 (9) 4417-4418; doi: 10.1073/pnas.97.9.4417.

[291] Lachenmeier DW: Wormwood (Artemisia absinthium L.)--a curious plant with both neurotoxic and neuroprotective properties? J Ethnopharmacol. 2010 Aug 19;131(1):224-7. doi: 10.1016/j.jep.2010.05.062.

[292] Abu-Darwish MS, Cabral C, Ferreira IV, et al. Essential oil of common sage (Salvia officinalis L.) from Jordan: assessment of safety in mammalian cells and its antifungal and anti-inflammatory potential. Biomed Res Int. 2013;2013:538940. doi: 10.1155/2013/538940.

[293] Lachenmeier DW, Uebelacker M: Risk assessment of thujone in foods and medicines containing sage and wormwood--evidence for a need of regulatory changes? Regul Toxicol Pharmacol. 2010 Dec;58(3):437-43. doi: 10.1016/j.yrtph.2010.08.012.

[294] del Castillo J, Anderson M, Rubottom GM: Marijuana, absinthe and the central nervous system. Nature. 1975 Jan 31;253(5490):365-6. PMID: 1110781.

[295] Höld KM, Sirisoma NS, Ikeda T, Narahashi T, Casida JE: Alpha-thujone (the active component of absinthe): gamma-aminobutyric acid type A receptor modulation and metabolic detoxification. Proc Natl Acad Sci U S A. 2000;97(8):3826-31. doi: 10.1073/pnas.070042397.

[296] Meschler JP, Howlett AC: Thujone exhibits low affinity for cannabinoid receptors but fails to evoke cannabimimetic responses. Pharmacol Biochem Behav. 1999 Mar;62(3):473-80. PMID: 10080239.

[297] Fernandes ES, Passos GF, Medeiros R, da Cunha FM, Ferreira J, Campos MM, Pianowski LF, Calixto JB: Anti-inflammatory effects of compounds alpha-humulene and (-)-trans-caryophyllene isolated from the essential oil of Cordia verbenacea. Eur J Pharmacol. 2007 Aug 27;569(3):228-36. doi: 10.1016/j.ejphar.2007.04.059.

[298] Schapowal, A, Klein, P, Johnston, SL: Echinacea reduces the risk of recurrent respiratory tract infections and complications: A meta-analysis of randomized controlled trials. Advances in Therapy. 32 (3): 187–200. doi:10.1007/s12325-015-0194-4.

[299] Gertsch J, Pertwee RG, Di Marzo V: Phytocannabinoids beyond the Cannabis plant - do they exist?. Br J Pharmacol. 2010;160(3):523-9. doi: 10.1111/j.1476-5381.2010.00745.x.

[300] Chicca A, Raduner S, Pellati F, Strompen T, Altmann KH, Schoop R, Gertsch J: Synergistic immunomopharmacological effects of N-alkylamides in Echinacea purpurea herbal extracts. Int Immunopharmacol. 2009 Jul; 9(7-8):850-8. doi: 10.1016/j.intimp.2009.03.006.

[301] Raduner S, Majewska A, Chen JZ, Xie XQ, Hamon J, Faller B, Altmann KH, Gertsch J: Alkylamides from Echinacea are a new class of cannabinomimetics. Cannabinoid type 2 receptor-dependent and -independent immunomodulatory effects. J Biol Chem. 2006 May 19;281(20):14192-206. doi: 10.1074/jbc.M601074200.

[302] Gertsch J, Schoop R, Kuenzle U, Suter A: Echinacea alkylamides modulate TNF-alpha gene expression via cannabinoid receptor CB2 and multiple signal transduction pathways. FEBS Lett. 2004 Nov 19;577(3):563-9. doi: 10.1016/j.febslet.2004.10.064.

[303] Nicolussi S, Viveros-Paredes JM, Gachet MS, Rau M, Flores-Soto ME, Blunder M, Gertsch J: Guineensine is a novel inhibitor of endocannabinoid uptake showing cannabimimetic behavioral effects in BALB/c mice. Pharmacol Res. 2014 Feb;80:52-65. doi: 10.1016/j.phrs.2013.12.010.

[304] Reynoso-Moreno I, Najar-Guerrero I, Escareño N, Flores-Soto ME, Gertsch J, Viveros-Paredes JM: An Endocannabinoid Uptake Inhibitor from Black Pepper Exerts Pronounced Anti-Inflammatory Effects in Mice. J Agric Food Chem. 2017 Nov 1;65(43):9435-9442. doi: 10.1021/acs.jafc.7b02979.

[305] Srinivasan K: Black pepper and its pungent principle-piperine: a review of diverse physiological effects. Crit Rev Food Sci Nutr. 2007;47(8):735-48. doi: 10.1080/10408390601062054.

[306] Han HK: The effects of black pepper on the intestinal absorption and hepatic metabolism of drugs. Expert Opin Drug Metab Toxicol. 2011 Jun;7(6):721-9. doi: 10.1517/17425255.2011.570332.

[307] Prakash UN, Srinivasan K: Beneficial influence of dietary spices on the ultrastructure and fluidity of the intestinal brush border in rats. Br J Nutr. 2010 Jul;104(1):31-9. doi: 10.1017/S0007114510000334.

[308] Khajuria A, Thusu N, Zutshi U: Piperine modulates permeability characteristics of intestine by inducing alterations in membrane dynamics: influence on brush border membrane fluidity, ultrastructure and enzyme kinetics. Phytomedicine. 2002 Apr;9(3):224-31. doi: 10.1078/0944-7113-00114.

[309] McNamara FN, Randall A, Gunthorpe MJ: Effects of piperine, the pungent component of black pepper, at the human vanilloid receptor (TRPV1). Br J Pharmacol. 2005 Mar;144(6):781-90. doi: 10.1038/sj.bjp.0706040.

[310] Majdalawieh AF, Carr RI: In vitro investigation of the potential immunomodulatory and anti-cancer activities of black pepper (Piper nigrum) and cardamom (Elettaria cardamomum). J Med Food. 2010 Apr;13(2):371-81. doi: 10.1089/jmf.2009.1131.

[311] Aravindaram K, Yang NS: Anti-inflammatory plant natural products for cancer therapy. Planta Med. 2010 Aug;76(11):1103-17. doi: 10.1055/s-0030-1249859.

[312] Butt MS, Pasha I, Sultan MT, Randhawa MA, Saeed F, Ahmed W: Black pepper and health claims: a comprehensive treatise. Crit Rev Food Sci Nutr. 2013;53(9):875-86. doi: 10.1080/10408398.2011.571799.

[313] Chavarria D, Silva T, Magalhães e Silva D, Remião F, Borges F: Lessons from black pepper: piperine and derivatives thereof. Expert Opin Ther Pat. 2016;26(2):245-64. doi: 10.1517/13543776.2016.1118057.

[314] Meghwal M, Goswami TK: Piper nigrum and piperine: an update. Phytother Res. 2013 Aug;27(8):1121-30. doi: 10.1002/ptr.4972.

[315] Bober Z, Stępień A, Aebisher D, Ożog L, Bartusik-Aebisher D: Medicinal benefits from the use of Black pepper, Curcuma and Ginger. Eur J Clin Exp Med 2018; 16 (2): 133–145. doi: 10.15584/ejcem.2018. 2.9.

[316] Barbaro B, Toietta G, Maggio R, et al: Effects of the olive-derived polyphenol oleuropein on human health. Int J Mol Sci. 2014;15(10): 18508-24. doi:10.3390/ijms151018508.

[317] Di Francesco A, Falconi A, Di Germanio C, Micioni Di Bonaventura MV, Costa A, Caramuta S, Del Carlo M, Compagnone D, Dainese E, Cifani C, Maccarrone M, D'Addario C: Extravirgin olive oil up-regulates CB1 tumor suppressor gene in human colon cancer cells and in rat colon via epigenetic mechanisms. J Nutr Biochem. 2015 Mar;26(3):250-8. doi: 10.1016/j.jnutbio.2014.10.013.

[318] Rigacci S, Stefani M: Nutraceutical Properties of Olive Oil Polyphenols. An Itinerary from Cultured Cells through Animal Models to Humans. Int J Mol Sci. 2016 May 31;17(6). pii: E843. doi: 10.3390/ijms17060843.

[319] Seely KA, Levi MS, Prather PL: The dietary polyphenols trans-resveratrol and curcumin selectively bind human CB1 cannabinoid receptors with nanomolar affinities and function as antagonists/inverse agonists. J Pharmacol Exp Ther. 2009 Jul;330(1):31-9. doi: 10.1124/jpet.109.151654.

[320] Thors L, Alajakku K, Fowler CJ: The 'specific' tyrosine kinase inhibitor genistein inhibits the enzymic hydrolysis of anandamide: implications for anandamide uptake. Br J Pharmacol. 2007;150(7):951-60. doi: 10.1038/sj.bjp.0707172.

[321] Thors L, Eriksson J, Fowler CJ: Inhibition of the cellular uptake of anandamide by genistein and its analogue daidzein in cells with different levels of fatty acid amide hydrolase-driven uptake. Br J Pharmacol. 2007 Nov;152(5):744-50. doi: 10.1038/sj.bjp.0707401.

[322] Thors L, Burston JJ, Alter BJ, McKinney MK, Cravatt BF, Ross RA, Pertwee RG, Gereau RW 4th, Wiley JL, Fowler CJ: Biochanin A, a naturally occurring inhibitor of fatty acid amide hydrolase. Br J Pharmacol. 2010 Jun;160(3):549-60. doi: 10.1111/j.1476-5381.2010.00716.x.

[323] McPartland JM, Guy GW, Di Marzo V: Care and feeding of the endocannabinoid system: a systematic review of potential clinical inter ventions that upregulate the endocannabinoid system. PLoS One. 2014 Mar 12;9(3):e89566.doi:10.1371/journal.pone.0089566. eCollection 2014.

[324] Dzhambazova E, Landzhov B, Malinova L, Kartelov Y, Abarova S: Increase In The Number Of Cb1 Immunopositive Neurons In The Amygdaloid Body After Acute Cold Stress Exposure. 106 Trakia Journal of Sciences, Vol. 12, Suppl. 1, 2014 Trakia Journal of Sciences, Vol. 12, Suppl. 1, pp 106-109, 2014.

[325] Krott LM, Piscitelli F, Heine M, Borrino S, Scheja L, Silvestri C, Heeren J, Di Marzo V: Endocannabinoid regulation in white and brown adipose tissue following thermogenic activation. J Lipid Res. 2016 Mar;57(3):464-73. doi: 10.1194/jlr.M065227.

[326] Rawls SM, Benamar K. Effects of opioids, cannabinoids, and vanilloids on body temperature. Front Biosci (Schol Ed). 2011;3:822–845. PMID: 21622235.

[327] Zhornitsky S, Potvin S. Cannabidiol in humans-the quest for therapeutic targets. Pharmaceuticals (Basel). 2012;5(5):529-52. doi:10.3390/ph5050529.

[328] McDonnell AM, Dang CH. Basic review of the cytochrome p450 system. J Adv Pract Oncol. 2013;4(4):263-8. PMID: 25032007.

[329] Bornheim LM, Grillo MP: Characterization of cytochrome P450 3A inactivation by cannabidiol: possible involvement of cannabidiol-hydroxyquinone as a P450 inactivator. Chem Res Toxicol. 1998 Oct;11(10):1209-16. doi: 10.1021/tx9800598.

[330] Yamaori S, Ebisawa J, Okushima Y, Yamamoto I, Watanabe K: Potent inhibition of human cytochrome P450 3A isoforms by cannabidiol: role of phenolic hydroxyl groups in the resorcinol moiety. Life Sci. 2011 Apr 11;88(15-16):730-6. doi: 10.1016/j.lfs.2011.02.017.

[331] Yamaori S, Kushihara M, Yamamoto I, Watanabe K: Characterization of major phytocannabinoids, cannabidiol and cannabinol, as isoform-selective and potent inhibitors of human CYP1 enzymes. Biochem Pharmacol. 2010 Jun 1;79(11):1691-8. doi: 10.1016/j.bcp.2010.01.028.

[332] Yamaori S, Okamoto Y, Yamamoto I, Watanabe K: Cannabidiol, a major phytocannabinoid, as a potent atypical inhibitor for CYP2D6. Drug Metab Dispos. 2011 Nov;39(11):2049-56. doi: 10.1124/dmd.111.041384.

[333] Yamaori S, Koeda K, Kushihara M, Hada Y, Yamamoto I, Watanabe K: Comparison in the in vitro inhibitory effects of major phytocannabinoids and polycyclic aromatic hydrocarbons contained in marijuana smoke on cytochrome P450 2C9 activity. Drug Metab Pharmacokinet. 2012;27(3):294-300. PMID: 22166891.

[334] Ohlsson A, Lindgren JE, Andersson S, Agurell S, Gillespie H, Hollister LE: Single-dose kinetics of deuterium-labelled cannabidiol in man after smoking and intravenous administration. Biomed Environ Mass Spectrom. 1986 Feb;13(2):77-83. PMID: 2937482.

[335] Huestis MA. Human cannabinoid pharmacokinetics. Chem Biodivers. 2007;4(8):1770-804. doi: 10.1002/cbdv.200790152.

[336] Ohlsson A, Lindgren JE, Wahlen A, Agurell S, Hollister LE, Gillespie HK: Plasma delta-9 tetrahydrocannabinol concentrations and clinical effects after oral and intravenous administration and smoking. Clin Pharmacol Ther. 1980 Sep;28(3):409-16. PMID: 6250760.

[337] Agurell S, Carlsson S, Lindgren JE, Ohlsson A, Gillespie H, Hollister L: Interactions of delta 1-tetrahydrocannabinol with cannabinol and cannabidiol following oral administration in man. Assay of cannabinol and cannabidiol by mass fragmentography. Experientia. 1981 Oct 15;37(10):1090-2. PMID: 6273208.

[338] Gronewold A, Skopp G: A preliminary investigation on the distribution of cannabinoids in man. Forensic Sci Int. 2011 Jul 15;210(1-3):e7-e11. doi: 10.1016/j.forsciint.2011.04.010..

[339] Alozie SO, Martin BR, Harris LS, Dewey WL: 3H-delta 9-Tetrahydrocannabinol, 3H-cannabinol and 3H-cannabidiol: penetration and regional distribution in rat brain. Pharmacol Biochem Behav. 1980 Feb;12(2):217-21. PMID: 6246544.

[340] Harvey DJ. Metabolism and pharmacokinetics of the cannabinoids. In: Biochemistry and physiology of substance abuse (Watson RR, editor, ed.). CRC Press: Boca Raton, 1991, pp. 279–365.

[341] Ujváry I, Hanuš L. Human Metabolites of Cannabidiol: A Review on Their Formation, Biological Activity, and Relevance in Therapy. Cannabis Cannabinoid Res. 2016;1(1):90–101. doi:10.1089/can.2015.0012.

[342] Harvey DJ, Samara E, Mechoulam R: Urinary metabolites of cannabidiol in dog, rat and man and their identification by gas chromatography-mass spectrometry. J Chromatogr. 1991 Jan 2;562(1-2):299-322. PMID: 2026700.

[343] Consroe P, Kennedy K, Schram K: Assay of plasma cannabidiol by capillary gas chromatography/ion trap mass spectroscopy following high-dose repeated daily oral administration in humans. Pharmacol Biochem Behav. 1991 Nov;40(3):517-22. PMID: 1666917.

[344] Devinsky O, Cilio MR, Cross H, Fernandez-Ruiz J, French J, Hill C, Katz R, Di Marzo V, Jutras-Aswad D, Notcutt WG, Martinez-Orgado J, Robson PJ, Rohrback BG, Thiele E, Whalley B, Friedman D. Cannabidiol: Pharmacology and potential therapeutic role in epilepsy and other neuropsychiatric disorders. Epilepsia. 2014; 55: 791–802. doi: 10.1111/epi.12631.

[345] Agurell S, Halldin M, Lindgren JE, Ohlsson A, Widman M, Gillespie H, Hollister L: Pharmacokinetics and metabolism of delta 1-tetrahydro cannabinol and other cannabinoids with emphasis on man. Pharmacol Rev. 1986 Mar;38(1):21-43. PMID: 3012605.

[346] Ohlsson A, Lindgren JE, Andersson S, Agurell S, Gillespie H, Hollister LE: Single-dose kinetics of deuterium-labelled cannabidiol in man after smoking and intravenous administration. Biomed Environ Mass Spectrom. 1986 Feb;13(2):77-83. PMID: 2937482.

[347] Wikipedia: Glia. en.wikipedia.org/wiki/Glia.

[348] Kozela E, Juknat A, Vogel Z. Modulation of Astrocyte Activity by Cannabidiol, a Nonpsychoactive Cannabinoid. Int J Mol Sci. 2017;18(8):1669. doi:10.3390/ijms18081669.

[349] Hind WH, England TJ, O'Sullivan SE: Cannabidiol protects an in vitro model of the blood-brain barrier from oxygen-glucose deprivation via PPARγ and 5-HT1A receptors. Br J Pharmacol. 2016 Mar;173(5):815-25. doi: 10.1111/bph.13368.

[350] Hind WH, Tufarelli C, Neophytou M, Anderson SI, England TJ, O'Sullivan SE: Endocannabinoids modulate human blood-brain barrier permeability in vitro. Br J Pharmacol. 2015 Jun;172(12):3015-27. doi: 10.1111/bph.13106.

[351] Campos AC, Fogaça MV, Sonego AB, Guimarães FS: Cannabidiol, neuroprotection and neuropsychiatric disorders. Pharmacol Res. 2016 Oct;112:119-127. doi: 10.1016/j.phrs.2016.01.033.

[352] Viveros MP, Marco EM, Llorente R, López-Gallardo M: Endocannabinoid system and synaptic plasticity: implications for emotional responses. Neural Plast. 2007;2007:52908. doi: 10.1155/2007/52908.

[353] Takeuchi T, Duszkiewicz AJ, Morris RG. The synaptic plasticity and memory hypothesis: encoding, storage and persistence. Philos Trans R Soc Lond B Biol Sci. 2014;369(1633):20130288. doi:10.1098/rstb.2013.0288.

[354] Martin SJ, Grimwood PD, Morris RG: Synaptic plasticity and memory: an evaluation of the hypothesis. Annu Rev Neurosci. 2000;23:649-711. doi: 10.1146/annurev.neuro.23.1.649.

[355] Love S, Plaha P, Patel NK, Hotton GR, BrooksDJ, Gill SS: Glial cell line–derived neurotrophic factor induces neuronal sprouting in human brain. Nature Medicine volume 11, pages 703–704 (2005). doi.org/10.1038/nm0705-703.

[356] Ben Achour S, Pascual O: Glia: the many ways to modulate synaptic plasticity. Neurochem Int. 2010 Nov;57(4):440-5. doi: 10.1016/j.neuint.2010.02.013.

[357] Mori MA, Meyer E, Soares LM, Milani H, Guimarães FS, de Oliveira RMW: Cannabidiol reduces neuroinflammation and promotes neuroplasticity and functional recovery after brain ischemia. Prog Neuropsychopharmacol Biol Psychiatry. 2017 Apr 3;75:94-105. doi: 10.1016/j.pnpbp.2016.11.005..

[358] Maren S, Baudry M: Properties and mechanisms of long-term synaptic plasticity in the mammalian brain: relationships to learning and memory. Neurobiol Learn Mem. 1995 Jan;63(1):1-18. doi: 10.1006/nlme.1995.1001

[359] Lee JLC, Bertoglio LJ, Guimarães FS, Stevenson CW. Cannabidiol regulation of emotion and emotional memory processing: relevance for treating anxiety-

related and substance abuse disorders. Br J Pharmacol. 2017;174(19):3242-3256. doi: 10.1111/bph.13724.

[360] Viveros MP, Marco EM, File SE: Endocannabinoid system and stress and anxiety responses. Pharmacol Biochem Behav. 2005 Jun;81(2):331-42. doi: 10.1016/j.pbb.2005.01.029.

[361] Jurkus R, Day HL, Guimarães FS, Lee JL, Bertoglio LJ, Stevenson CW: Cannabidiol Regulation of Learned Fear: Implications for Treating Anxiety-Related Disorders. Front Pharmacol. 2016 Nov 24;7:454 . doi: 10.3389/fphar.2016.00454.

[362] Marco EM, Viveros MP: Functional role of the endocannabinoid system in emotional homeostasis. Rev Neurol. 2009 Jan 1-15;48(1):20-6. PMID: 19145562.

[363] Defining the Human Microbiome. Nutr Rev. 2012 Aug; 70(Suppl 1): S38–S44. doi: 10.1111/j.1753-4887.2012.00493.x.

[364] The human microbiome project. Nature. 2007 Oct 18;449(7164):804-10. doi: 10.1038/nature06244.

[365] Microbial co-occurrence relationships in the human microbiome. PLoS Comput Biol. 2012;8(7):e1002606. doi: 10.1371/journal.pcbi.1002606.

[366] The microbiome as a human organ. Clin Microbiol Infect. 2012 Jul;18 Suppl 4:2-4. doi: 10.1111/j.1469-0691.2012.03916.x.

[367] NIH Human Microbiome Project defines normal bacterial makeup of the body. www.nih.gov/news-events/news-releases/nih-human-microbiome-project-defines-normal-bacterial-makeup-body.

[368] Metagenomic Analysis of the Human Distal Gut Microbiome. Science. 2006 Jun 2; 312(5778): 1355–1359. doi: 10.1126/science.1124234.

[369] A human gut microbial gene catalogue established by metagenomic sequencing. Nature volume 464, 2010: pages 59–65.

[370] Finishing the euchromatic sequence of the human genome. Nature. 2004 Oct 21;431(7011):931-45. doi: 10.1038/nature03001.

[371] Defining the Human Microbiome. Nutr Rev. 2012 Aug; 70(Suppl 1): S38–S44. doi: 10.1111/j.1753-4887.2012.00493.x.

[372] Ochoa-Cortes F, Turco F, Linan-Rico A, et al. Enteric Glial Cells: A New Frontier in Neurogastroenterology and Clinical Target for Inflammatory Bowel Diseases. Inflamm Bowel Dis. 2015;22(2):433-49. doi: 10.1097/MIB.0000000000000667.

[373] Izzo AA: Cannabinoids and intestinal motility: welcome to CB2 receptors. Br J Pharmacol. 2004 Aug;142(8):1201-2. doi: 10.1038/sj.bjp.0705890.

[374] Coutts AA, Izzo AA: The gastrointestinal pharmacology of cannabinoids: an update. Curr Opin Pharmacol. 2004 Dec;4(6):572-9. doi: 10.1016/j.coph.2004.05.007.

[375] Duncan M, Mouihate A, Mackie K, et al. Cannabinoid CB2 receptors in the enteric nervous system modulate gastrointestinal contractility in lipopolysaccharide-treated rats. Am J Physiol Gastrointest Liver Physiol. 2008;295(1):G78-G87. doi: 10.1152/ajpgi.90285.2008.

[376] Izzo AA: The cannabinoid CB(2) receptor: a good friend in the gut. Neurogastroenterol Motil. 2007 Sep;19(9):704-8. doi: 10.1111/j.1365-2982.2007.00977.x.

377 Cani PD, Plovier H, Van Hul M, Geurts L, Delzenne NM, Druart C, Everard A: Endocannabinoids--at the crossroads between the gut microbiota and host metabolism. Nat Rev Endocrinol. 2016 Mar;12(3) :133-43. doi: 10.1038/nrendo.2015.211.

378 Singh RK, Chang HW, Yan D, et al. Influence of diet on the gut microbiome and implications for human health. J Transl Med. 2017;15(1):73. doi:10.1186/s12967-017-1175-y.

379 Duda-Chodak A, Tarko T, Satora P, Sroka P: Interaction of dietary compounds, especially polyphenols, with the intestinal microbiota: a review. Eur J Nutr. 2015 Apr;54(3):325-41. doi: 10.1007/s00394-015-0852-y.

380 Muccioli GG, Naslain D, Bäckhed F, Reigstad CS, Lambert DM, Delzenne NM, Cani PD: The endocannabinoid system links gut microbiota to adipogenesis. Mol Syst Biol. 2010 Jul;6:392. doi: 10.1038/msb.2010.46.

381 DiPatrizio NV. Endocannabinoids in the Gut. Cannabis Cannabinoid Res. 2016;1(1):67-77. doi: 10.1089/can.2016.0001.

382 Wright KL, Duncan M, Sharkey KA. Cannabinoid CB2 receptors in the gastrointestinal tract: a regulatory system in states of inflammation. Br J Pharmacol. 2007;153(2):263-70. doi: 10.1038/sj.bjp.0707486.

383 e Filippis D, Esposito G, Cirillo C, Cipriano M, De Winter BY, Scuderi C, Sarnelli G, Cuomo R, Steardo L, De Man JG, Iuvone T: Cannabidiol reduces intestinal inflammation through the control of neuroimmune axis. PLoS One. 2011;6(12):e28159. doi: 10.1371/journal.pone.0028159.

384 Ahmed W, Katz S. Therapeutic Use of Cannabis in Inflammatory Bowel Disease. Gastroenterol Hepatol (N Y). 2016;12(11):668-679. PMID: 28035196.

385 Esposito G, Filippis DD, Cirillo C, Iuvone T, Capoccia E, Scuderi C, Steardo A, Cuomo R, Steardo L: Cannabidiol in inflammatory bowel diseases: a brief overview. Phytother Res. 2013 May;27(5):633-6. doi: 10.1002/ptr.4781.

386 Sharkey KA, Darmani NA, Parker LA: Regulation of nausea and vomiting by cannabinoids and the endocannabinoid system. Eur J Pharmacol. 2014 Jan 5;722:134-46. doi: 10.1016/j.ejphar.2013.09.068.

387 Sticht MA, Rock EM, Limebeer CL, Parker LA: Endocannabinoid Mechanisms Influencing Nausea. Int Rev Neurobiol. 2015;125:127-62. doi: 10.1016/bs.irn.2015.09.001.

388 Sharkey KA, Wiley JW. The Role of the Endocannabinoid System in the Brain-Gut Axis. Gastroenterology. 2016;151(2):252-66. doi: 10.1053/j.gastro.2016.04.015.

389 Sticht MA, Limebeer CL, Rafla BR, Parker LA: Intra-visceral insular cortex 2-arachidonoylglycerol, but not N-arachidonoylethanolamide, suppresses acute nausea-induced conditioned gaping in rats. Neuroscience. 2015 Feb 12;286:338-44. doi: 10.1016/j.neuroscience. 2014.11.058.

390 Sampson TR, Debelius JW, Thron T, Janssen S, Shastri GG, Ilhan ZE, Challis C, Schretter CE, Rocha S, Gradinaru V, Chesselet MF, Keshavarzian A, Shannon KM, Krajmalnik-Brown R, Wittung-Stafshede P, Knight R, Mazmanian SK: Gut Microbiota Regulate Motor Deficits and Neuroinflammation in a Model of Parkinson's Disease. Cell. 2016 Dec 1;167(6):1469-1480.e12. doi: 10.1016/j.cell.2016.11.018.

[391] He M, Shi B: Gut microbiota as a potential target of metabolic syndrome: the role of probiotics and prebiotics. Cell Biosci. 2017 Oct 25;7:54. doi: 10.1186/s13578-017-0183-1. doi: 10.1186/s13578-017-0183-1.

[392] Palermo FA, Mosconi G, Avella MA, Carnevali O, Verdenelli MC, Cecchini C, Polzonetti-Magni AM: Modulation of cortisol levels, endocannabinoid receptor 1A, proopiomelanocortin and thyroid hormone receptor alpha mRNA expressions by probiotics during sole (Solea solea) larval development. Gen Comp Endocrinol. 2011 May 1;171(3):293-300. doi: 10.1016/j.ygcen.2011.02.009.

[393] Zuardi AW, Guimarães FS, Moreira AC: Effect of cannabidiol on plasma prolactin, growth hormone and cortisol in human volunteers. Braz J Med Biol Res. 1993 Feb;26(2):213-7. PMID: 8257923.

[394] Watanabe K, Motoya E, Matsuzawa N, Funahashi T, Kimura T, Matsunaga T, Arizono K, Yamamoto I: Marijuana extracts possess the effects like the endocrine disrupting chemicals. Toxicology. 2005 Jan 31;206(3):471-8. doi: 10.1016/j.tox.2004.08.005.

[395] Rosenkrantz H, Esber HJ: Cannabinoid-induced hormone changes in monkeys and rats. J Toxicol Environ Health. 1980 Mar;6(2):297-313. doi: 10.1080/15287398009529853.

[396] List A, Nazar B, Nyquist S, Harclerode J: The effects of delta9-tetrahydrocannabinol and cannabidiol on the metabolism of gonadal steroids in the rat. Drug Metab Dispos. 1977 May-Jun;5(3):268-72. PMID: 17525.

[397] Gruden G, Barutta F, Kunos G, Pacher P. Role of the endocannabinoid system in diabetes and diabetic complications. Br J Pharmacol. 2015;173(7):1116-27. doi: 10.1111/bph.13226.

[398] Jadoon KA, Ratcliffe SH, Barrett DA, Thomas EL, Stott C, Bell JD, O'Sullivan SE, Tan GD: Efficacy and Safety of Cannabidiol and Tetrahydrocannabivarin on Glycemic and Lipid Parameters in Patients With Type 2 Diabetes: A Randomized, Double-Blind, Placebo-Controlled, Parallel Group Pilot Study. Diabetes Care. 2016 Oct;39(10):1777-86. doi: 10.2337/dc16-0650.

[399] Jamaluddin MS, Weakley SM, Yao Q, Chen C. Resistin: functional roles and therapeutic considerations for cardiovascular disease. Br J Pharmacol. 2012;165(3):622-32. doi:10.1111/j.1476-5381.2011.01369.x.

[400] Brellenthin AG, Crombie KM, Hillard CJ, Koltyn KF: Endocannabinoid and Mood Responses to Exercise in Adults with Varying Activity Levels. Med Sci Sports Exerc. 2017 Aug;49(8):1688-1696. doi: 10.1249/MSS.0000000000001276.

[401] Ware MA, Jensen D, Barrette A, Vernec A, Derman W. Cannabis and the Health and Performance of the Elite Athlete. Clin J Sport Med. 2018; 28(5):480–484. doi:10.1097/JSM.0000000000000650.

[402] Kennedy MC: Cannabis: Exercise performance and sport. A systematic review. J Sci Med Sport. 2017 Sep;20(9):825-829. doi: 10.1016/j.jsams.2017.03.012.

[403] Raichlen DA, Foster AD, Gerdeman GL, Seillier A, Giuffrida A: Wired to run: exercise-induced endocannabinoid signaling in humans and cursorial mammals with implications for the 'runner's high'. J Exp Biol. 2012 Apr 15;215(Pt 8):1331-6. doi: 10.1242/jeb.063677.

[404] Raichlen DA, Foster AD, Seillier A, Giuffrida A, Gerdeman GL: Exercise-induced endocannabinoid signaling is modulated by intensity. Eur J Appl Physiol. 2013 Apr;113(4):869-75. doi: 10.1007/s00421-012-2495-5.

[405] Meyer JD, Crombie KM, Cook DB Hillard CJ, Koltyn KF: Serum Endocannabinoid and Mood Changes after Exercise in Major Depressive Disorder. Med Sci Sports Exerc. 2019 Apr 8. doi: 10.1249/MSS.0000000000002006.

[406] de Mello Schier AR, de Oliveira Ribeiro NP, Coutinho DS, Machado S, Arias-Carrión O, Crippa JA, Zuardi AW, Nardi AE, Silva AC: Antidepressant-like and anxiolytic-like effects of cannabidiol: a chemical compound of Cannabis sativa. CNS Neurol Disord Drug Targets. 2014;13(6):953-60. PMID: 24923339.

[407] Schier AR, Ribeiro NP, Silva AC, Hallak JE, Crippa JA, Nardi AE, Zuardi AW: Cannabidiol, a Cannabis sativa constituent, as an anxiolytic drug. Braz J Psychiatry. 2012 Jun;34 Suppl 1:S104-10. PMID: 22729452.

[408] Gomes da Silva S, Araujo BH, Cossa AC, Scorza FA, Cavalheiro EA, Naffah-Mazzacoratti Mda G, Arida RM: Physical exercise in adolescence changes CB1 cannabinoid receptor expression in the rat brain. Neurochem Int. 2010 Nov;57(5):492-6. doi: 10.1016/j.neuint.2010.07.001.

[409] Yan ZC, Liu DY, Zhang LL, Shen CY, Ma QL, Cao TB, Wang LJ, Nie H, Zidek W, Tepel M, Zhu ZM: Exercise reduces adipose tissue via cannabinoid receptor type 1 which is regulated by peroxisome proliferator-activated receptor-delta. Biochem Biophys Res Commun. 2007 Mar 9;354(2):427-33. doi: 10.1016/j.bbrc.2006.12.213.

[410] James PT: Obesity: the worldwide epidemic. Clin Dermatol. 2004 Jul-Aug;22(4):276-80. doi: 10.1016/j.clindermatol.2004.01.010.

[411] James PT, Leach R, Kalamara E, Shayeghi M: The worldwide obesity epidemic. Obes Res. 2001 Nov;9 Suppl 4:228S-233S. doi: 10.1038/oby.2001.123.

[412] Hruby A, Hu FB: The Epidemiology of Obesity: A Big Picture. Pharma coeconomics. 2015;33(7):673-89. doi: 10.1007/s40273-014-0243-x.

[413] National Institute of health NIH: What is Prevalence? www.nimh.nih.gov/health/statistics/what-is-prevalence.shtml.

[414] Flegal KM, Carroll MD, Ogden CL, Johnson CL: Prevalence and trends in obesity among US adults, 1999-2000. JAMA 2002;288:1723-1727. PMID: 12365955.

[415] Stevens GA, Singh GM, Lu Y, Danaei G, Lin JK, Finucane MM, Bahalim AN, McIntire RK, Gutierrez HR, Cowan M, Paciorek CJ, Farzadfar F, Riley L, Ezzati M, Global Burden of Metabolic Risk Factors of Chronic Diseases Collaborating Group (Body Mass Index): National, regional, and global trends in adult overweight and obesity prevalences. Popul Health Metr. 2012 Nov 20;10(1):22. doi: 10.1186/1478-7954-10-22.

[416] Wang Y, Beydoun MA, Liang L, Caballero B, Kumanyika SK: Will all Americans become overweight or obese? estimating the progression and cost of the US obesity epidemic. Obesity (Silver Spring). 2008 Oct;16(10):2323-30. doi: 10.1038/oby.2008.351.

[417] Ogden CL, Carroll MD1, Kit BK2, Flegal KM1: Prevalence of childhood and adult obesity in the United States, 2011-2012. JAMA. 2014 Feb 26;311(8):806-14. doi: 10.1001/jama.2014.732.

[418] Olshansky SJ, Passaro DJ, Hershow RC, Layden J, Carnes BA, Brody J, Hayflick L, Butler RN, Allison DB, Ludwig DS: A potential decline in life expectancy in the United States in the 21st century. N Engl J Med. 2005 Mar 17;352(11):1138-45. doi: 10.1056/NEJMsr043743.

[419] Horn H, Böhme B, Dietrich L, Koch M: Endocannabinoids in Body Weight Control. Pharmaceuticals (Basel). 2018 May 30;11(2). pii: E55. doi: 10.3390/ph11020055.

[420] Fride E, Ginzburg Y, Breuer A, Bisogno T, Di Marzo V, Mechoulam R: Critical role of the endogenous cannabinoid system in mouse pup suckling and growth. Eur J Pharmacol. 2001 May 11;419(2-3):207-14. PMID: 11426843.

[421] Aguirre CA, Castillo VA, Llanos MN: Excess of the endocannabinoid anandamide during lactation induces overweight, fat accumulation and insulin resistance in adult mice. Diabetol Metab Syndr. 2012 Jul 23;4(1):35. doi: 10.1186/1758-5996-4-35.

[422] Aguirre CA, Castillo VA, Llanos MN: The endocannabinoid anandamide during lactation increases body fat content and CB1 receptor levels in mice adipose tissue. Nutr Diabetes. 2015 Jun 22;5:e167. doi: 10.1038/nutd.2015.17.

[423] Di Marzo V, Piscitelli F, Mechoulam R: Cannabinoids and endocannabinoids in metabolic disorders with focus on diabetes. Handb Exp Pharmacol. 2011;(203):75-104. doi: 10.1007/978-3-642-17214-4_4.

[424] Giralt M, Villarroya F: White, brown, beige/brite: different adipose cells for different functions? Endocrinology. 2013 Sep;154(9):2992-3000. doi: 10.1210/en.2013-1403.

[425] Park A, Kim WK, Bae KH: Distinction of white, beige and brown adipocytes derived from mesenchymal stem cells. World J Stem Cells. 2014 Jan 26;6(1):33-42. doi: 10.4252/wjsc.v6.i1.33.

[426] Cereijo R, Giralt M, Villarroya F: Thermogenic brown and beige/brite adipogenesis in humans. Ann Med. 2015 Mar;47(2):169-77. doi: 10.3109/07853890.2014.952328.

[427] McMillan AC, White MD: Induction of thermogenesis in brown and beige adipose tissues: molecular markers, mild cold exposure and novel therapies. Curr Opin Endocrinol Diabetes Obes. 2015 Oct;22(5):347-52. doi: 10.1097/MED.0000000000000191.

[428] Krott LM, Piscitelli F, Heine M, Borrino S, Scheja L, Silvestri C, Heeren J, Di Marzo V: Endocannabinoid regulation in white and brown adipose tissue following thermogenic activation. J Lipid Res. 2016 Mar;57(3):464-73. doi: 10.1194/jlr.M065227.

[429] Parray HA, Yun JW: Cannabidiol promotes browning in 3T3-L1 adipocytes. Mol Cell Biochem. 2016 May;416(1-2):131-9. doi: 10.1007/s11010-016-2702-5.

[430] Kim SH, Plutzky J: Brown Fat and Browning for the Treatment of Obesity and Related Metabolic Disorders. Diabetes Metab J. 2016 Feb;40(1):12-21. doi: 10.4093/dmj.2016.40.1.12.

431 Corroon J, Phillips JA. A Cross-Sectional Study of Cannabidiol Users. Cannabis Cannabinoid Res. 2018;3(1):152–161. Published 2018 Jul 1. doi:10.1089/can.2018.0006.

432 Brochstein A: Study Shows CBD is Replacing Traditional Pharmaceuticals. New Cannabis Ventures 2017. www.newcannabisventures.com/study-shows-cbd-is-replacing-traditional-pharmaceuticals.

433 The world health report 2002 - reducing risks, promoting healthy life. World Health Organization WHO.

434 World Health Organization WHO. Fact Sheets. Mental disorders. www.who.int/news-room/fact-sheets/detail/mental-disorders.

435 FDA News Release:FDA approves first drug comprised of an active ingredient derived from marijuana to treat rare, severe forms of epilepsy. fda.gov/newsevents/newsroom/pressannouncements/ucm611046.htm.

436 Devinsky O, Marsh E, Friedman D, Thiele E, Laux L, Sullivan J, Miller, Flamini R, Wilfong A, Filloux F, Wong M, Tilton N, Bruno P, Bluvstein J, Hedlund J, Kamens R, Maclean J, Nangia S, Singhal NS, Wilson CA, Patel A, Cilio MR: Cannabidiol in patients with treatment-resistant epilepsy: an open-label interventional trial. Lancet Neurol. 2016 Mar;15(3):270-8. doi: 10.1016/S1474-4422(15)00379-8.

437 Reithmeier D, Tang-Wai R, Seifert B, Lyon AW, Alcorn J, Acton B, Corley S, Prosser-Loose E, Mousseau DD, Lim HJ, Tellez-Zenteno J, Huh L, Leung E, Carmant L, Huntsman RJ: The protocol for the Cannabidiol in children with refractory epileptic encephalopathy (CARE-E) study: a phase 1 dosage escalation study. BMC Pediatr. 2018 Jul 7;18(1):221. doi: 10.1186/s12887-018-1191-y.

438 Devinsky O, Cilio MR, Cross H, Fernandez-Ruiz J, French J, Hill C, Katz R, Di Marzo V, Jutras-Aswad D, Notcutt WG, Martinez-Orgado J, Robson PJ, Rohrback BG, Thiele E, Whalley B, Friedman D: Cannabidiol: pharmacology and potential therapeutic role in epilepsy and other neuropsychiatric disorders. Epilepsia. 2014 Jun;55(6):791-802. doi: 10.1111/epi.12631.

439 Campos AC, Moreira FA, Gomes FV, Del Bel EA, Guimarães FS: Multiple mechanisms involved in the large-spectrum therapeutic potential of cannabidiol in psychiatric disorders. Philos Trans R Soc Lond B Biol Sci. 2012 Dec 5;367(1607):3364-78. doi: 10.1098/rstb.2011.0389.

440 Hayakawa K, Mishima K, Fujiwara M. Therapeutic Potential of Non-Psychotropic Cannabidiol in Ischemic Stroke. Pharmaceuticals (Basel). 2010;3(7):2197–2212. doi:10.3390/ph3072197.

441 Zuardi AW, Crippa JA, Hallak JE, Moreira FA, Guimarães FS: Cannabidiol, a Cannabis sativa constituent, as an antipsychotic drug. Braz J Med Biol Res. 2006 Apr;39(4):421-9. doi: /S0100-879X2006000400001.

442 Deiana S: Medical use of cannabis. Cannabidiol: a new light for schizo phrenia? Drug Test Anal. 2013 Jan;5(1):46-51. doi: 10.1002/dta.1425.

443 Watt G, Karl T. In vivo Evidence for Therapeutic Properties of Cannabidiol (CBD) for Alzheimer's Disease. Front Pharmacol. 2017;8:20. doi:10.3389/fphar.2017.00020.

444 Dementia Care Central: Using CBD (Cannabidiol) to Treat the Symptoms of Alzheimer's & Other Dementias. www.dementiacarecentral.com/aboutdementia/treating/cbd.

[445] Karl T, Cheng D, Garner B, Arnold JC: The therapeutic potential of the endocannabinoid system for Alzheimer's disease. Expert Opinion on Therapeutic Targets. Volume 16, 2012 - Issue 4. doi.org/10.1517/14728222.2012.671812.

[446] Karl T, Garner B, Cheng D: The therapeutic potential of the phytocannabinoid cannabidiol for Alzheimer's disease. Behav Pharmacol. 2017 Apr;28(2 and 3-Spec Issue):142-160. doi: 10.1097/FBP.0000000000000247.

[447] Kyle SD, Morgan K, Espie CA: Insomnia and health-related quality of life. Sleep Med Rev. 2010 Feb;14(1):69-82. doi: 10.1016/j.smrv.2009.07.004.

[448] Hossain JL, Shapiro CM: The prevalence, cost implications, and management of sleep disorders: an overview. Sleep Breath. 2002 Jun;6(2):85-102. doi: 10.1007/s11325-002-0085-1.

[449] Ferrie JE, Kumari M, Salo P, Singh-Manoux A, Kivimäki M. Sleep epidemiology--a rapidly growing field. Int J Epidemiol. 2011;40(6):1431–1437. doi:10.1093/ije/dyr203.

[450] Pava MJ, Makriyannis A2, Lovinger DM: Endocannabinoid Signaling Regulates Sleep Stability. PLoS One. 2016 Mar 31;11(3):e0152473. doi: 10.1371/journal.pone.0152473.

[451] Shannon S, Lewis N, Lee H, Hughes S: Cannabidiol in Anxiety and Sleep: A Large Case Series. Perm J. 2019;23:18–041. doi:10.7812/TPP/18-041.

[452] Babson KA, Sottile J, Morabito D: Cannabis, Cannabinoids, and Sleep: a Review of the Literature. Curr Psychiatry Rep. 2017 Apr;19(4):23. doi: 10.1007/s11920-017-0775-9.

[453] Chagas MH, Crippa JA, Zuardi AW, Hallak JE, Machado-de-Sousa JP, Hirotsu C, Maia L, Tufik S, Andersen ML: Effects of acute systemic administration of cannabidiol on sleep-wake cycle in rats. J Psychopharmacol. 2013 Mar;27(3):312-6. doi: 10.1177/0269881112474524.

[454] Shannon S, Opila-Lehman J: Effectiveness of Cannabidiol Oil for Pediatric Anxiety and Insomnia as Part of Posttraumatic Stress Disorder: A Case Report. Perm J. 2016 Fall;20(4):16-005. doi: 10.7812/TPP/16-005.

[455] Linares IMP, Guimaraes FS, Eckeli A, et al. No Acute Effects of Cannabidiol on the Sleep-Wake Cycle of Healthy Subjects: A Randomized, Double-Blind, Placebo-Controlled, Crossover Study. Front Pharmacol. 2018;9:315. doi:10.3389/fphar.2018.00315.

[456] Murillo-Rodríguez E, Millán-Aldaco D, Palomero-Rivero M, Mechoulam R, Drucker-Colín R: Cannabidiol, a constituent of Cannabis sativa, modulates sleep in rats. FEBS Lett. 2006 Aug 7;580(18):4337-45. doi: 10.1016/j.febslet.2006.04.102.

[457] Carlini EA, Cunha JM: Hypnotic and antiepileptic effects of cannabidiol. J Clin Pharmacol.1981 Aug-Sep;21(S1):417S-427S.PMID:7028792.

[458] Babson KA, Sottile J, Morabito D: Cannabis, Cannabinoids, and Sleep: a Review of the Literature. Curr Psychiatry Rep (2017) 19: 23. doi.org/10.1007/s11920-017-0775-9.

[459] Bandelow B, Michaelis S. Epidemiology of anxiety disorders in the 21st century. Dialogues Clin Neurosci. 2015;17(3):327–335.

[460] Kessler RC, Ruscio AM, Shear K, Wittchen HU. Epidemiology of anxiety disorders. Curr Top Behav Neurosci. 2010;2:21-35. PMID: 21309104.

461 Schier AR, Ribeiro NP, Silva AC, Hallak JE, Crippa JA, Nardi AE, Zuardi AW: Cannabidiol, a Cannabis sativa constituent, as an anxiolytic drug. Braz J Psychiatry. 2012 Jun;34 Suppl 1:S104-10. PMID: 22729452.

462 Soares VP, Campos AC. Evidences for the Anti-panic Actions of Cannabidiol. Curr Neuropharmacol. 2017;15(2):291–299. doi:10.2174/1570159X14666160509123955.

463 Crippa JA, Derenusson GN, Ferrari TB, Wichert-Ana L, Duran FL, Martin-Santos R, Simões MV, Bhattacharyya S, Fusar-Poli P, Atakan Z, Santos Filho A, Freitas-Ferrari MC, McGuire PK, Zuardi AW, Busatto GF, Hallak JE: Neural basis of anxiolytic effects of cannabidiol (CBD) in generalized social anxiety disorder: a preliminary report. J Psychopharmacol. 2011 Jan;25(1):121-30. doi: 10.1177/0269881110379283.

464 Blessing EM, Steenkamp MM, Manzanares J, Marmar CR: Cannabidiol as a Potential Treatment for Anxiety Disorders. Neurotherapeutics. 2015 Oct;12(4):825-36. doi: 10.1007/s13311-015-0387-1.

465 de Mello Schier AR, de Oliveira Ribeiro NP, Coutinho DS, Machado S, Arias-Carrión O, Crippa JA, Zuardi AW, Nardi AE, Silva AC: Antidepressant-like and anxiolytic-like effects of cannabidiol: a chemical compound of Cannabis sativa. CNS Neurol Disord Drug Targets. 2014;13(6):953-60. PMID: 24923339.

466 Gomes FV, Resstel LB, Guimarães FS: The anxiolytic-like effects of cannabidiol injected into the bed nucleus of the stria terminalis are mediated by 5-HT1A receptors. Psychopharmacology (Berl). 2011 Feb;213(2-3):465-73. doi: 10.1007/s00213-010-2036-z.

467 Lee JLC, Bertoglio LJ, Guimarães FS, Stevenson CW: Cannabidiol regulation of emotion and emotional memory processing: relevance for treating anxiety-related and substance abuse disorders. Br J Pharmacol. 2017 Oct;174(19):3242-3256. doi: 10.1111/bph.13724.

468 Jurkus R, Day HL, Guimarães FS, Lee JL, Bertoglio LJ, Stevenson CW: Cannabidiol Regulation of Learned Fear: Implications for Treating Anxiety-Related Disorders. Front Pharmacol. 2016 Nov 24;7:454. eCollection 2016. doi: 10.3389/fphar.2016.00454.

469 Lee JLC, Bertoglio LJ, Guimarães FS, Stevenson CW: Cannabidiol regulation of emotion and emotional memory processing: relevance for treating anxiety-related and substance abuse disorders. Br J Pharmacol. 2017 Oct;174(19):3242-3256. doi: 10.1111/bph.13724.

470 Zuardi AW, Cosme RA, Graeff FG, Guimarães FS: Effects of ipsapirone and cannabidiol on human experimental anxiety. J Psychopharmacol. 1993 Jan;7(1 Suppl):82-8. doi: 10.1177/026988119300700112.

471 Bergamaschi MM, Queiroz RH, Chagas MH, de Oliveira DC, De Martinis BS, Kapczinski F, Quevedo J, Roesler R, Schröder N, Nardi AE, Martín-Santos R, Hallak JE, Zuardi AW, Crippa JA: Cannabidiol reduces the anxiety induced by simulated public speaking in treatment-naïve social phobia patients. Neuropsychopharmacology. 2011 May;36(6):1219-26. doi: 10.1038/npp.2011.6.

472 St Sauver JL, Warner DO, Yawn BP, et al. Why patients visit their doctors: assessing the most prevalent conditions in a defined American population. Mayo Clin Proc. 2013;88(1):56–67. doi:10.1016/j.mayocp.2012.08.020.

[473] Deyo RA, Mirza SK, Martin BI: Back pain prevalence and visit rates: estimates from U.S. national surveys, 2002. Spine (Phila Pa 1976). 2006 Nov 1;31(23):2724-7. doi: 10.1097/01.brs.0000244618.06877.cd.

[474] Hart LG, Deyo RA, Cherkin DC: Physician office visits for low back pain. Frequency, clinical evaluation, and treatment patterns from a U.S. national survey. Spine (Phila Pa 1976). 1995 Jan 1;20(1):11-9. PMID: 7709270.

[475] Nahin RL: Estimates of pain prevalence and severity in adults: United States, 2012. J Pain. 2015 Aug;16(8):769-80. doi: 10.1016/j.jpain.2015.05.002.

[476] Russo EB. Cannabinoids in the management of difficult to treat pain. Ther Clin Risk Manag. 2008;4(1):245–259. PMID: 18728714.

[477] Britch SC, Wiley JL, Yu Z, Clowers BH, Craft RM: Cannabidiol-Δ9-tetrahydrocannabinol interactions on acute pain and locomotor activity. Drug Alcohol Depend. 2017 Jun 1;175:187-197. doi: 10.1016/j.drugalcdep.2017.01.046.

[478] Rahn EJ, Makriyannis A, Hohmann AG: Activation of cannabinoid CB1 and CB2 receptors suppresses neuropathic nociception evoked by the chemotherapeutic agent vincristine in rats. Br J Pharmacol. 2007 Nov;152(5):765-77. doi: 10.1038/sj.bjp.0707333.

[479] Costa B, Giagnoni G, Franke C, Trovato AE, Colleoni M: Vanilloid TRPV1 receptor mediates the antihyperalgesic effect of the nonpsychoactive cannabinoid, cannabidiol, in a rat model of acute inflammation. Br J Pharmacol. 2004 Sep;143(2):247-50. doi: 10.1038/sj.bjp.0705920.

[480] Miller RJ, Miller RE: Is cannabis an effective treatment for joint pain? Clin Exp Rheumatol. 2017 Sep-Oct;35 Suppl 107(5):59-67.

[481] Manzanares J, Julian M, Carrascosa A. Role of the cannabinoid system in pain control and therapeutic implications for the management of acute and chronic pain episodes. Curr Neuropharmacol. 2006;4(3):239–257.

[482] Xiong W, Cui T, Cheng K, et al. Cannabinoids suppress inflammatory and neuropathic pain by targeting α3 glycine receptors. J Exp Med. 2012;209(6):1121–1134. doi:10.1084/jem.20120242.

[483] Mücke M, Phillips T, Radbruch L, Petzke F, Häuser W: Cannabis-based medicines for chronic neuropathic pain in adults. Cochrane Database Syst Rev. 2018 Mar 7;3:CD012182. doi: 10.1002/14651858.CD012182.pub2.

[484] Hammell DC, Zhang LP, Ma F, et al. Transdermal cannabidiol reduces inflammation and pain-related behaviours in a rat model of arthritis. Eur J Pain. 2015;20(6):936–948. doi:10.1002/ejp.818.

[485] Wade DT, Robson P, House H, Makela P, Aram J: A preliminary controlled study to determine whether whole-plant cannabis extracts can improve intractable neurogenic symptoms. Clin Rehabil. 2003 Feb;17(1):21-9. doi: 10.1191/0269215503cr581oa.

[486] Liput DJ, Hammell DC, Stinchcomb AL, Nixon K: Transdermal delivery of cannabidiol attenuates binge alcohol-induced neurodegeneration in a rodent model of an alcohol use disorder. Pharmacol Biochem Behav. 2013 Oct;111:120-7. doi: 10.1016/j.pbb.2013.08.013.

[487] Hammell DC, Zhang LP, Ma F, Abshire SM, McIlwrath SL, Stinchcomb AL, Westlund KN: Transdermal cannabidiol reduces inflammation and pain-related behaviours in a rat model of arthritis. Eur J Pain. 2016 Jul;20(6):936-48. doi: 10.1002/ejp.818.

[488] Malfait AM, Gallily R, Sumariwalla PF, Malik AS, Andreakos E, Mechoulam R, Feldmann M: The nonpsychoactive cannabis constituent cannabidiol is an oral anti-arthritic therapeutic in murine collagen-induced arthritis. Proc Natl Acad Sci U S A. 2000 Aug 15;97(17):9561-6. doi: 10.1073/pnas.160105897.

[489] Ward SJ, McAllister SD, Kawamura R, Murase R, Neelakantan H, Walker EA: Cannabidiol inhibits paclitaxel-induced neuropathic pain through 5-HT(1A) receptors without diminishing nervous system function or chemotherapy efficacy. Br J Pharmacol. 2014 Feb;171(3):636-45. doi: 10.1111/bph.12439.

[490] Chuong CM, Nickoloff BJ, Elias PM, Goldsmith LA, Macher E, Maderson PA, Sundberg JP, Tagami H, Plonka PM, Thestrup-Pederson K, Bernard BA, Schröder JM, Dotto P, Chang CM, Williams ML, Feingold KR, King LE, Kligman AM, Rees JL, Christophers E: What is the 'true' function of skin? Exp Dermatol. 2002 Apr;11(2):159-87. PMID: 11994143.

[491] Neill US. Skin care in the aging female: myths and truths. J Clin Invest. 2012;122(2):473–477. doi:10.1172/JCI61978.

[492] Ganceviciene R, Liakou AI, Theodoridis A, Makrantonaki E, Zouboulis CC. Skin anti-aging strategies. Dermatoendocrinol. 2012;4(3):308–319. doi:10.4161/derm.22804.

[493] Facial symmetry and judgements of apparent health: support for a 'good genes' explanation of the attractiveness–symmetry relationship. Evol. Hum. Behav. 22, 417–42910.1016/S1090-5138(01)00083-6. doi:10.1016/S1090-5138(01)00083-6.

[494] Bíró T, Tóth BI, Haskó G, Paus R, Pacher P. The endocannabinoid system of the skin in health and disease: novel perspectives and therapeutic opportunities. Trends Pharmacol Sci. 2009;30(8):411–420. doi:10.1016/j.tips.2009.05.004.

[495] Roosterman D, Goerge T, Schneider SW, Bunnett NW, Steinhoff M: Neuronal control of skin function: the skin as a neuroimmunoendocrine organ. Physiol Rev. 2006 Oct;86(4):1309-79. doi: 10.1152/physrev.00026.2005

[496] Lotti T, Hautmann G, Panconesi E: Neuropeptides in skin. J Am Acad Dermatol. 1995 Sep;33(3):482-96. PMID: 7657872

[497] Tóth KF, Ádám D, Bíró T, Oláh A. Cannabinoid Signaling in the Skin: Therapeutic Potential of the "C(ut)annabinoid" System. Molecules. 2019;24(5):918. doi:10.3390/molecules24050918

[498] Sánchez-Carpintero I, España-Alonso A: Role of neuropeptides in dermatology. Rev Neurol. 1997 Sep;25 Suppl 3:S222-31. PMID: 9273166.

[499] Denda M: Newly discovered olfactory receptors in epidermal keratinocytes are associated with proliferation, migration, and re-epithelialization of keratinocytes. J Invest Dermatol. 2014 Nov;134(11):2677-2679. doi: 10.1038/jid.2014.229.

[500] Shaw L, Mansfield C, Colquitt L, Lin C, Ferreira J, Emmetsberger J, Reed DR: Personalized expression of bitter 'taste' receptors in human skin. PLoS One. 2018 Oct 17;13(10):e0205322. doi: 10.1371/journal.pone.0205322.

[501] Gilca M, Dragos D. Extraoral Taste Receptor Discovery: New Light on Ayurvedic Pharmacology. Evid Based Complement Alternat Med. 2017;2017:5435831. doi:10.1155/2017/5435831.

[502] Zheng JL, Yu TS, Li XN, Fan YY, Ma WX, Du Y, Zhao R, Guan D: Cannabinoid receptor type 2 is time-dependently expressed during skin wound healing in mice. Int J Legal Med. 2012 Sep;126(5):807-14. doi: 10.1007/s00414-012-0741-3.

[503] Russo EB. Taming THC: potential cannabis synergy and phytocannabinoid-terpenoid entourage effects. Br J Pharmacol. 2011;163(7):1344-64. doi: 10.1111/j.1476-5381.2011.01238.x.

[504] Oláh A, Tóth BI, Borbíró I, Sugawara K, Szöllõsi AG, Czifra G, Pál B, Ambrus L, Kloepper J, Camera E, Ludovici M, Picardo M, Voets T, Zouboulis CC, Paus R, Bíró T: Cannabidiol exerts sebostatic and antiinflammatory effects on human sebocytes. J Clin Invest. 2014 Sep;124(9):3713-24. doi: 10.1172/JCI64628.

[505] Namdar D, Koltai H: Medical Cannabis for the Treatment of Inflammation. Natural Product Information 2018. Volume: 13 issue: 3. doi.org/10.1177/1934578X1801300304.

[506] Wilkinson JD, Williamson E: Cannabinoids inhibit human keratinocyte proliferation through a non-CB1/CB2 mechanism and have a potential therapeutic value in the treatment of psoriasis. J Dermatol Sci. 2007 Feb;45(2):87-92. 10.1016/j.jdermsci.2006.10.009.

[507] Oláh A, Markovics A, Szabó-Papp J, Szabó PT, Stott C, Zouboulis CC, Bíró T: Differential effectiveness of selected non-psychotropic phytocannabinoids on human sebocyte functions implicates their introduction in dry/seborrhoeic skin and acne treatment. Exp Dermatol. 2016 Sep;25(9):701-7. doi: 10.1111/exd.13042.

[508] Paul R, Williams R, Hodson V, Peake C. Detection of cannabinoids in hair after cosmetic application of hemp oil. Sci Rep. 2019;9(1):2582. Published 2019 Feb 22. doi:10.1038/s41598-019-39609-0.

[509] Mercati F, Dall'Aglio C, Pascucci L, Boiti C, Ceccarelli P: Identification of cannabinoid type 1 receptor in dog hair follicles. Acta Histochem. 2012 Jan;114(1):68-71. doi: 10.1016/j.acthis.2011.01.003.

[510] Telek A, Bíró T, Bodó E, Tóth BI, Borbíró I, Kunos G, Paus R: FASEB J. 2007 Nov;21(13):3534-41. doi: 10.1096/fj.06-7689com.

[511] Bodó E, Bíró T, Telek A, Czifra G, Griger Z, Tóth BI, Mescalchin A, Ito T, Bettermann A, Kovács L, Paus R: A hot new twist to hair biology: involvement of vanilloid receptor-1 (VR1/TRPV1) signaling in human hair growth control. Am J Pathol. 2005 Apr;166(4):985-98. doi: 10.1016/S0002-9440(10)62320-6.

[512] Borbíró I, Lisztes E, Tóth BI, Czifra G, Oláh A, Szöllosi AG, Szentandrássy N, Nánási PP, Péter Z, Paus R, Kovács L, Bíró T: Activation of transient receptor potential vanilloid-3 inhibits human hair growth. J Invest Dermatol. 2011 Aug;131(8):1605-14. doi: 10.1038/jid.2011.122.

[513] Inci R, Kelekci KH, Oguz N, Karaca S, Karadas B, Bayrakci A: Dermatological aspects of synthetic cannabinoid addiction. Cutan Ocul Toxicol. 2017 Jun;36(2):125-131. doi: 10.3109/15569527.2016.1169541.

[514] Pucci M, Pasquariello N, Battista N, et al. Endocannabinoids stimulate human melanogenesis via type-1 cannabinoid receptor. J Biol Chem. 2012;287(19):15466–15478. doi:10.1074/jbc.M111.314880.

[515] Pacioni G, Rapino C, Zarivi O, Falconi A, Leonardi M, Battista N, Colafarina S, Sergi M, Bonfigli A, Miranda M, Barsacchi D, Maccarrone M: Truffles contain

endocannabinoid metabolic enzymes and anandamide. Phytochemistry. 2015 Feb;110:104-10. doi: 10.1016/j.phytochem.2014.11.012.

[516] Caterina MJ. TRP channel cannabinoid receptors in skin sensation, homeostasis, and inflammation. ACS Chem Neurosci. 2014;5(11):1107–1116. doi:10.1021/cn5000919.

[517] Stamberger J: Medical Marijuana Inc, News: Study Finds CBD-Based Topical Improves Skin Appearance. 2016; news.medicalmarijuana inc.com/study-finds-cbd-based-topical-improves-skin-appearance.

[518] Heron M, Anderson RN: Changes in the Leading Cause of Death: Recent Patterns in Heart Disease and Cancer Mortality. NCHS Data Brief. 2016 Aug;(254):1-8. PMID: 27598767.

[519] Global, regional, and national life expectancy, all-cause mortality, and cause-specific mortality for 249 causes of death, 1980-2015: a systematic analysis for the Global Burden of Disease Study 2015. GBD 2015 Mortality and Causes of Death Collaborators. Lancet. 2016 Oct 8; 388(10053):1459-1544. doi: 10.1016/S0140-6736(16)31012-1.

[520] Nagai H, Kim YH. Cancer prevention from the perspective of global cancer burden patterns. J Thorac Dis. 2017;9(3):448–451. doi:10.21037/jtd.2017.02.75. doi: 10.21037/jtd.2017.02.75.

[521] Sarfaraz S, Adhami VM, Syed DN, Afaq F, Mukhtar H: Cannabinoids for cancer treatment: progress and promise. Cancer Res. 2008 Jan 15;68(2):339-42. doi: 10.1158/0008-5472.CAN-07-2785.

[522] Chakravarti B, Ravi J, Ganju RK. Cannabinoids as therapeutic agents in cancer: current status and future implications. Oncotarget. 2014;5(15):5852–5872. doi:10.18632/oncotarget.2233.

[523] Joseph J, Niggemann B, Zaenker KS, Entschladen F: Anandamide is an endogenous inhibitor for the migration of tumor cells and T lymphocytes. Cancer Immunol Immunother. 2004 Aug;53(8):723-8. doi: 10.1007/s00262-004-0509-9.

[524] Śledziński P, Zeyland J, Słomski R, Nowak A. The current state and future perspectives of cannabinoids in cancer biology [published correction appears in Cancer Med. 2018 Nov;7(11):5859]. Cancer Med. 2018;7(3):765–775. doi:10.1002/cam4.1312.

[525] De Petrocellis L, Melck D, Palmisano A, Bisogno T, Laezza C, Bifulco M, Di Marzo V: The endogenous cannabinoid anandamide inhibits human breast cancer cell proliferation. Proc Natl Acad Sci U S A. 1998 Jul 7;95(14):8375-80. PMID: 9653194.

[526] Blázquez C, Carracedo A, Barrado L, Real PJ, Fernández-Luna JL, Velasco G, Malumbres M, Guzmán M: Cannabinoid receptors as novel targets for the treatment of melanoma. FASEB J. 2006 Dec;20(14):2633-5. doi: 10.1096/fj.06-6638fje.

[527] Caffarel MM, Andradas C, Mira E, Pérez-Gómez E, Cerutti C, Moreno-Bueno G, Flores JM, García-Real I, Palacios J, Mañes S, Guzmán M, Sánchez C: Cannabinoids reduce ErbB2-driven breast cancer progression through Akt inhibition. Mol Cancer. 2010 Jul 22;9:196. doi: 10.1186/1476-4598-9-196. doi: 10.1186/1476-4598-9-196.

[528] Sarfaraz S, Afaq F, Adhami VM, Mukhtar H: Cannabinoid receptor as a novel target for the treatment of prostate cancer. Cancer Res. 2005 Mar 1;65(5):1635-41. doi: 10.1158/0008-5472.CAN-04-3410.

[529] Ramer R, Hinz B: Cannabinoids as Anticancer Drugs. Adv Pharmacol. 2017;80:397-436. doi: 10.1016/bs.apha.2017.04.002.

[530] Donadelli M, Dando I, Zaniboni T, et al. Gemcitabine/cannabinoid combination triggers autophagy in pancreatic cancer cells through a ROS-mediated mechanism. Cell Death Dis. 2011;2(4):e152. doi:10.1038/cddis.2011.36.

[531] Massi P, Vaccani A, Ceruti S, Colombo A, Abbracchio MP, Parolaro D: Antitumor effects of cannabidiol, a nonpsychoactive cannabinoid, on human glioma cell lines. J Pharmacol Exp Ther. 2004 Mar;308(3):838-45. doi: 10.1124/jpet.103.061002.

[532] Shen Y, Lu Y, Yu F, Zhu C, Wang H, Wang J: Peroxisome Proliferator-Activated Receptor-γ and Its Ligands in the Treatment of Tumors in the Nervous System. Curr Stem Cell Res Ther. 2016;11(3):208-15. PMID: 26216127.

[533] Ramer R, Heinemann K, Merkord J, Rohde H, Salamon A, Linnebacher M, Hinz B: COX-2 and PPAR-γ confer cannabidiol-induced apoptosis of human lung cancer cells. Mol Cancer Ther. 2013 Jan;12(1):69-82. doi: 10.1158/1535-7163.MCT-12-0335.

[534] Bisogno T, Hanus L, De Petrocellis L, Tchilibon S, Ponde DE, Brandi I, Moriello AS, Davis JB, Mechoulam R, Di Marzo V: Molecular targets for cannabidiol and its synthetic analogues: effect on vanilloid VR1 receptors and on the cellular uptake and enzymatic hydrolysis of anandamide. Br J Pharmacol. 2001 Oct;134(4):845-52. doi: 10.1038/sj.bjp.0704327.

[535] Ravi J, Sneh A, Shilo K, Nasser MW, Ganju RK: FAAH inhibition enhances anandamide mediated anti-tumorigenic effects in non-small cell lung cancer by downregulating the EGF/EGFR pathway. Oncotarget. 2014 May 15;5(9):2475-86. doi: 10.18632/oncotarget.1723.

[536] Aggarwal SK. Use of cannabinoids in cancer care: palliative care. Curr Oncol. 2016;23(2):S33–S36. doi:10.3747/co.23.2962.

[537] Abrams DI, Guzman M: Cannabis in cancer care. Clin Pharmacol Ther. 2015 Jun;97(6):575-86. doi: 10.1002/cpt.108.

[538] Dzierżanowski T. Prospects for the Use of Cannabinoids in Oncology and Palliative Care Practice: A Review of the Evidence. Cancers (Basel). 2019;11(2):129. doi:10.3390/cancers11020129.

[539] Tateo S: State of the evidence: Cannabinoids and cancer pain—A systematic review. Journal of the American Association of Nurse Practitioners 2017. 29(2):94–103, doi: 10.1002/2327-6924.12422.

[540] Tramèr MR, Carroll D, Campbell FA, Reynolds DJ, Moore RA, McQuay HJ: Cannabinoids for control of chemotherapy induced nausea and vomiting: quantitative systematic review. BMJ. 2001 Jul 7;323(7303):16-21. PMID: 11440936.

[541] Cooper GS, Stroehla BC: The epidemiology of autoimmune diseases. Autoimmun Rev. 2003 May;2(3):119-25. PMID: 12848952

[542] Cooper GS, Bynum ML, Somers EC. Recent insights in the epidemiology of autoimmune diseases: improved prevalence estimates and understanding of

clustering of diseases. J Autoimmun. 2009;33(3-4):197–207. doi:10.1016/j.jaut.2009.09.008.

[543] Jacobson DL, Gange SJ, Rose NR, Graham NM: Epidemiology and estimated population burden of selected autoimmune diseases in the United States. Clin Immunol Immunopathol. 1997 Sep;84(3):223-43. PMID: 9281381.

[544] Qin X. What caused the increase of autoimmune and allergic diseases: a decreased or an increased exposure to luminal microbial components? World J Gastroenterol. 2007;13(8):1306–1307. doi:10.3748/wjg.v13.i8.1306.

[545] Cojocaru M, Cojocaru IM, Silosi I. Multiple autoimmune syndrome. Maedica (Buchar). 2010;5(2):132–134.

[546] Hewagama A, Richardson B: The genetics and epigenetics of autoimmune diseases. J Autoimmun. 2009 Aug;33(1):3-11. doi: 10.1016/j.jaut.2009.03.007.

[547] Katchan V, David P, Shoenfeld Y: Cannabinoids and autoimmune diseases: A systematic review. Autoimmun Rev. 2016 Jun;15(6):513-28. doi: 10.1016/j.autrev.2016.02.008.

[548] Rieder SA, Chauhan A, Singh U, Nagarkatti M, Nagarkatti P: Cannabinoid-induced apoptosis in immune cells as a pathway to immunosuppression. Immunobiology. 2010 Aug;215(8):598-605. doi: 10.1016/j.imbio.2009.04.001.

[549] Pandey R, Hegde VL, Singh NP, Hofseth L, Singh U, Ray S, Nagarkatti M, Nagarkatti PS: Use of cannabinoids as a novel therapeutic modality against autoimmune hepatitis. Vitam Horm. 2009;81:487-504. doi: 10.1016/S0083-6729(09)81019-4.

[550] Hegde VL, Hegde S, Cravatt BF, Hofseth LJ, Nagarkatti M, Nagarkatti PS: Attenuation of experimental autoimmune hepatitis by exogenous and endogenous cannabinoids: involvement of regulatory T cells. Mol Pharmacol. 2008 Jul;74(1):20-33. doi: 10.1124/mol.108.047035.

[551] Arévalo-Martín A, García-Ovejero D, Gómez O, Rubio-Araiz A, Navarro-Galve B, Guaza C, Molina-Holgado E, Molina-Holgado F: CB2 cannabinoid receptors as an emerging target for demyelinating diseases: from neuroimmune interactions to cell replacement strategies. Br J Pharmacol. 2008 Jan;153(2):216-25. doi: 10.1038/sj.bjp.0707466.

[552] Weiner HL: The challenge of multiple sclerosis: how do we cure a chronic heterogeneous disease? Ann Neurol. 2009 Mar;65(3):239-48. doi: 10.1002/ana.21640.

[553] Nagarkatti P, Pandey R, Rieder SA, Hegde VL, Nagarkatti M. Cannabinoids as novel anti-inflammatory drugs. Future Med Chem. 2009;1(7):1333–1349. doi:10.4155/fmc.09.93.

[554] Elliott DM, Singh N, Nagarkatti M, Nagarkatti PS. Cannabidiol Attenuates Experimental Autoimmune Encephalomyelitis Model of Multiple Sclerosis Through Induction of Myeloid-Derived Suppressor Cells. Front Immunol. 2018;9:1782. 2018 doi:10.3389/fimmu.2018.01782.

[555] Kozela E, Lev N, Kaushansky N, Eilam R, Rimmerman N, Levy R, Ben-Nun A, Juknat A, Vogel Z: Cannabidiol inhibits pathogenic T cells, decreases spinal microglial activation and ameliorates multiple sclerosis-like disease in C57BL/6 mice. Br J Pharmacol. 2011 Aug;163(7):1507-19. doi: 10.1111/j.1476-5381.2011.01379.x.

[556] Rahimi A, Faizi M, Talebi F, Noorbakhsh F, Kahrizi F, Naderi N: Interaction between the protective effects of cannabidiol and palmitoylethanolamide in

experimental model of multiple sclerosis in C57BL/6 mice. Neuroscience. 2015 Apr 2;290:279-87. doi: 10.1016/j.neuroscience.2015.01.030.

[557] Kaplan BL, Springs AE, Kaminski NE. The profile of immune modulation by cannabidiol (CBD) involves deregulation of nuclear factor of activated T cells (NFAT). Biochem Pharmacol. 2008;76(6):726–737. doi:10.1016/j.bcp.2008.06.022.

[558] Weiss L, Zeira M, Reich S, Har-Noy M, Mechoulam R, Slavin S, Gallily R: Cannabidiol lowers incidence of diabetes in non-obese diabetic mice. Autoimmunity. 2006 Mar;39(2):143-51. doi: 10.1080/08916930500356674.

[559] Katz D, Katz I, Porat-Katz BS, Shoenfeld Y: Medical cannabis: Another piece in the mosaic of autoimmunity? Clin Pharmacol Ther. 2017 Feb;101(2):230-238. doi: 10.1002/cpt.568.

[560] Mechoulam R, Parker LA, Gallily R: Cannabidiol: an overview of some pharmacological aspects. J Clin Pharmacol. 2002 Nov;42(S1):11S-19S. PMID: 12412831.

[561] Hammell DC, Zhang LP, Ma F, et al. Transdermal cannabidiol reduces inflammation and pain-related behaviours in a rat model of arthritis. Eur J Pain. 2015;20(6):936–948. doi:10.1002/ejp.818.

[562] De Filippis D, Esposito G, Cirillo C, Cipriano M, De Winter BY, Scuderi C, Sarnelli G, Cuomo R, Steardo L, De Man JG, Iuvone T: Cannabidiol reduces intestinal inflammation through the control of neuroimmune axis. PLoS One. 2011;6(12):e28159. doi: 10.1371/journal.pone.0028159.

[563] Li B, Selmi C, Tang R, Gershwin ME, Ma X: The microbiome and autoimmunity: a paradigm from the gut-liver axis. Cell Mol Immunol. 2018 Jun;15(6):595-609. doi: 10.1038/cmi.2018.7.

[564] De Luca F, Shoenfeld Y: The microbiome in autoimmune diseases. Clin Exp Immunol. 2019 Jan;195(1):74-85. doi: 10.1111/cei.13158.

[565] Cani PD, Plovier H, Van Hul M, Geurts L, Delzenne NM, Druart C, Everard A: Endocannabinoids--at the crossroads between the gut microbiota and host metabolism. Nat Rev Endocrinol. 2016 Mar;12(3):133-43. doi: 10.1038/nrendo.2015.211.

[566] Sözen T, Özışık L, Başaran NÇ: An overview and management of osteoporosis. Eur J Rheumatol. 2017 Mar;4(1):46-56. doi: 10.5152/eurjrheum.2016.048.

[567] International Osteoporosis Foundation. Osteoporosis- Incidence and burden. www.iofbonehealth.org/facts-statistics.

[568] Johnell O, Kanis JA: An estimate of the worldwide prevalence and disability associated with osteoporotic fractures. Osteoporos Int. 2006 Dec;17(12):1726-33. doi: 10.1007/s00198-006-0172-4.

[569] Kanis JA, Johnell O, De Laet C, Johansson H: A meta-analysis of previous fracture and subsequent fracture risk. Bone. 2004 Aug;35(2):375-82. doi: 10.1016/j. bone.2004.03.024.

[570] Ofek O, Karsak M, Leclerc N, Fogel M, Frenkel B, Wright K, Tam J, Attar-Namdar M, Kram V, Shohami E, Mechoulam R, Zimmer A, Bab I: Peripheral cannabinoid receptor, CB2, regulates bone mass. Proc Natl Acad Sci U S A. 2006 Jan 17;103(3):696-701. doi: 10.1073/pnas.0504187103

[571] Idris AI, Sophocleous A, Landao-Bassonga E, van't Hof RJ, Ralston SH: Regulation of bone mass, osteoclast function, and ovariectomy-induced bone

loss by the type 2 cannabinoid receptor. Endocrinology. 2008 Nov;149(11):5619-26. doi: 10.1210/en.2008-0150.

[572] Bab I, Zimmer A, Melamed E: Cannabinoids and the skeleton: from marijuana to reversal of bone loss. Ann Med. 2009;41(8):560-7. doi: 10.1080/07853890903121025.

[573] Kogan NM, Melamed E, Wasserman E, Raphael B, Breuer A, Stok KS, Sondergaard R, Escudero AV, Baraghithy S, Attar-Namdar M, Friedlander-Barenboim S, Mathavan N, Isaksson H, Mechoulam R, Müller R, Bajayo A, Gabet Y, Bab I: Cannabidiol, a Major Non-Psychotropic Cannabis Constituent Enhances Fracture Healing and Stimulates Lysyl Hydroxylase Activity in Osteoblasts. J Bone Miner Res. 2015 Oct;30(10):1905-13. doi: 10.1002/jbmr.2513.

[574] Li D, Lin Z, Meng Q, Wang K, Wu J, Yan H: Cannabidiol administration reduces sublesional cancellous bone loss in rats with severe spinal cord injury. Eur J Pharmacol. 2017 Aug 15;809:13-19. doi: 10.1016/j.ejphar.2017.05.011.

[575] Marino S, Idris AI: Emerging therapeutic targets in cancer induced bone disease: A focus on the peripheral type 2 cannabinoid receptor. Pharmacol Res. 2017 May;119:391-403. doi: 10.1016/j.phrs.2017.02.023.

[576] MacDonald S, Hall J. Bone pain. In: MacDonald N, Oneschuk D, Hagen N, Doyle D, editors. Palliative medicine: a case-based manual. 2. New York, NY: Oxford University Press; 2005. pp. 47–58.

[577] Tam J, Trembovler V, Di Marzo V, Petrosino S, Leo G, Alexandrovich A, Regev E, Casap N, Shteyer A, Ledent C, Karsak M, Zimmer A, Mechoulam R, Yirmiya R, Shohami E, Bab I: The cannabinoid CB1 receptor regulates bone formation by modulating adrenergic signaling. FASEB J. 2008 Jan;22(1):285-94. doi: 10.1096/fj.06-7957com.

[578] Heron M, Anderson RN: Changes in the Leading Cause of Death: Recent Patterns in Heart Disease and Cancer Mortality. NCHS Data Brief. 2016 Aug;(254):1-8. PMID: 27598767.

[579] Gaziano T, Reddy KS, Paccaud F, Horton S, Chaturvedi V: Disease Control Priorities in Developing Countries. 2nd edition. Chapter 33, Cardiovascular Disease. www.ncbi.nlm.nih.gov/books/NBK11767/ Co-published by Oxford University Press, New York.

[580] Anand SS, Hawkes C, de Souza RJ, et al. Food Consumption and its Impact on Cardiovascular Disease: Importance of Solutions Focused on the Globalized Food System: A Report From the Workshop Convened by the World Heart Federation. J Am Coll Cardiol. 2015;66(14):1590–1614. doi:10.1016/j.jacc.2015.07.050.

[581] Rippe JM, Angelopoulos TJ: Lifestyle strategies for cardiovascular risk reduction. Curr Atheroscler Rep. 2014 Oct;16(10):444. doi: 10.1007/s11883-014-0444-y.

[582] Masana L, Ros E, Sudano I, Angoulvant D; lifestyle expert working group: Is there a role for lifestyle changes in cardiovascular prevention? What, when and how? Atheroscler Suppl. 2017 Apr;26:2-15. doi: 10.1016/S1567-5688(17)30020-X.

[583] Lake KD, Compton DR, Varga K, Martin BR, Kunos G: Cannabinoid-induced hypotension and bradycardia in rats mediated by CB1-like cannabinoid receptors. J Pharmacol Exp Ther. 1997 Jun;281(3):1030-7. PMID: 9190833.

[584] Martín Giménez VM, Noriega SE, Kassuha DE, Fuentes LB, Manucha W: Anandamide and endocannabinoid system: an attractive therapeutic approach for cardiovascular disease. Ther Adv Cardiovasc Dis. 2018 Jul;12(7):177-190. doi: 10.1177/1753944718773690.

[585] O'Sullivan SE: Endocannabinoids and the Cardiovascular System in Health and Disease. Handb Exp Pharmacol. 2015;231:393-422. doi: 10.1007/978-3-319-20825-1_14.

[586] Grainger J, Boachie-Ansah G. Anandamide-induced relaxation of sheep coronary arteries: the role of the vascular endothelium, arachidonic acid metabolites and potassium channels. Br J Pharmacol. 2001;134(5):1003–1012. doi:10.1038/sj.bjp.0704340.

[587] Steffens S, Pacher P: The activated endocannabinoid system in atherosclerosis: driving force or protective mechanism? Curr Drug Targets. 2015;16(4):334-41. PMID: 25469884.

[588] Montecucco F, Di Marzo V: At the heart of the matter: the endocannabinoid system in cardiovascular function and dysfunction. Trends Pharmacol Sci. 2012 Jun;33(6):331-40. doi: 10.1016/j.tips.2012.03.002.

[589] Cook C, Foster P: Epidemiology of glaucoma: what's new? Can J Ophthalmol. 2012 Jun;47(3):223-6. doi: 10.1016/j.jcjo.2012.02.003.

[590] Straiker AJ, Maguire G, Mackie K, Lindsey J: Localization of cannabinoid CB1 receptors in the human anterior eye and retina. Invest Ophthalmol Vis Sci. 1999 Sep;40(10):2442-8. PMID: 10476817.

[591] Hepler RS, Frank IR: Marihuana smoking and intraocular pressure. JAMA. 1971 Sep 6;217(10):1392. PMID: 5109652.

[592] Tomida I, Pertwee RG, Azuara-Blanco A. Cannabinoids and glaucoma. Br J Ophthalmol. 2004;88(5):708–713. doi:10.1136/bjo.2003.032250.

[593] Korczyn AD: The ocular effects of cannabinoids. General Pharmacology: The Vascular System. Volume 11, Issue 5, 1980, Pages 419-423. doi.org/10.1016/0306-3623(80)90026-9.

[594] Järvinen T, Pate DW, Laine K: Cannabinoids in the treatment of glaucoma. Pharmacol Ther. 2002 Aug;95(2):203-20. PMID: 12182967.

[595] Nucci C, Bari M, Spanò A, Corasaniti M, Bagetta G, Maccarrone M, Morrone LA: Potential roles of (endo)cannabinoids in the treatment of glaucoma: from intraocular pressure control to neuroprotection. Prog Brain Res. 2008;173:451-64. doi: 10.1016/S0079-6123(08)01131-X.

[596] Kelly B, Nappe T: National Center for Biotechnology Information NCBI. StatPearls: Cannabinoid Toxicity. ncbi.nlm.nih.gov/books/NBK482175/.

[597] Huecker MR, Azadfard M, Leaming JM: Opioid Addiction. [Updated 2019 Feb 28]. In: StatPearls [Internet]. StatPearls Publishing; 2019. Available from: www.ncbi.nlm.nih.gov/books/NBK448203.

[598] Hser YI, Mooney LJ, Saxon AJ, et al. High Mortality Among Patients With Opioid Use Disorder in a Large Healthcare System. J Addict Med. 2017;11(4):315–319. doi:10.1097/ADM.0000000000000312.

[599] Gomes T, Tadrous M, Mamdani MM, Paterson JM, Juurlink DN. The Burden of Opioid-Related Mortality in the United States. JAMA Netw Open. 2018;1(2):e180217. Published 2018 Jun 1. doi:10.1001/jamanetworkopen.2018.0217.

[600] Rudd RA, Seth P, David F, Scholl L: Increases in Drug and Opioid-Involved Overdose Deaths - United States, 2010-2015. MMWR Morb Mortal Wkly Rep. 2016 Dec 30;65(50-51):1445-1452. doi: 10.15585/mmwr.mm655051e1.

[601] Centers for disease Control and Prevention Understanding the Epidemic. Record Overdose Deaths. cdc.gov/drugoverdose/epidemic/index.

[602] Prud'homme M, Cata R, Jutras-Aswad D. Cannabidiol as an Intervention for Addictive Behaviors: A Systematic Review of the Evidence. Subst Abuse. 2015;9:33–38. doi:10.4137/SART.S25081.

[603] Katsidoni V, Anagnostou I, Panagis G: Cannabidiol inhibits the reward-facilitating effect of morphine: involvement of 5-HT1A receptors in the dorsal raphe nucleus. Addict Biol. 2013 Mar;18(2):286-96. doi: 10.1111/j.1369-1600.2012.00483.x.

[604] Ren Y, Whittard J, Higuera-Matas A, Morris CV, Hurd YL: Cannabidiol, a nonpsychotropic component of cannabis, inhibits cue-induced heroin seeking and normalizes discrete mesolimbic neuronal disturbances. J Neurosci. 2009 Nov 25;29(47):14764-9. doi: 10.1523/JNEUROSCI.4291-09.2009.

[605] Crippa JA, Hallak JE, Machado-de-Sousa JP, Queiroz RH, Bergamaschi M, Chagas MH, Zuardi AW: Cannabidiol for the treatment of cannabis withdrawal syndrome: a case report. J Clin Pharm Ther. 2013 Apr;38(2):162-4. doi: 10.1111/jcpt.12018.

[606] Morgan CJ, Schafer G, Freeman TP, Curran HV: Impact of cannabidiol on the acute memory and psychotomimetic effects of smoked cannabis: naturalistic study: naturalistic study. Br J Psychiatry. 2010 Oct;197(4):285-90. doi: 10.1192/bjp.bp.110.077503.

[607] Morgan CJ, Freeman TP, Schafer GL, Curran HV: Cannabidiol attenuates the appetitive effects of Delta 9-tetrahydrocannabinol in humans smoking their chosen cannabis. Neuropsychopharmacology. 2010 Aug;35(9):1879-85. doi: 10.1038/npp.2010.58.

[608] Morgan CJ, Das RK, Joye A, Curran HV, Kamboj SK: Cannabidiol reduces cigarette consumption in tobacco smokers: preliminary findings. Addict Behav. 2013 Sep;38(9):2433-6. doi: 10.1016/j.addbeh.2013.03.011.

[609] Consroe P, Carlini EA, Zwicker AP, Lacerda LA: Interaction of cannabidiol and alcohol in humans. Psychopharmacology (Berl). 1979;66(1):45-50. PMID: 120541.

[610] Turna J, Syan SK, Frey BN, Rush B, Costello MJ, Weiss M, MacKillop J: Cannabidiol as a Novel Candidate Alcohol Use Disorder Pharmacotherapy: A Systematic Review. Alcohol Clin Exp Res. 2019 Apr;43(4):550-563. doi: 10.1111/acer.13964.

[611] Bradford AC, Bradford WD, Abraham A, Bagwell Adams G: Association Between US State Medical Cannabis Laws and Opioid Prescribing in the Medicare Part D Population. JAMA Intern Med. 2018;178(5):667–672.

[612] Corroon J, Phillips JA. A Cross-Sectional Study of Cannabidiol Users. Cannabis Cannabinoid Res. 2018;3(1):152–161. doi:10.1089/can.2018.0006.

[613] Iffland K, Grotenhermen F. An Update on Safety and Side Effects of Cannabidiol: A Review of Clinical Data and Relevant Animal Studies. Cannabis Cannabinoid Res. 2017;2(1):139–154. doi:10.1089/can.2016.0034.

[614] The U.S. Food and Drug Administration FDA: Scientific Data and Information about Products Containing Cannabis or Cannabis-Derived

Compounds; Public Hearing. May 2019. www.fda.gov/news-events/fda-meetings-conferences-and-workshops/scientific-data-and-information-about-products-containing-cannabis-or-cannabis-derived-compounds.

[615] Jiang R, Yamaori S, Okamoto Y, Yamamoto I, Watanabe K: Cannabidiol is a potent inhibitor of the catalytic activity of cytochrome P450 2C19. Drug Metab Pharmacokinet. 2013;28(4):332-8. PMID: 23318708.

[616] Yamaori S, Okamoto Y, Yamamoto I, Watanabe K: Cannabidiol, a major phytocannabinoid, as a potent atypical inhibitor for CYP2D6. Drug Metab Dispos. 2011 Nov;39(11):2049-56. doi: 10.1124/dmd.111.041384.

[617] Rong C, Carmona NE, Lee YL, Ragguett RM, Pan Z, Rosenblat JD, Subramaniapillai M, Shekotikhina M, Almatham F, Alageel A, Mansur R, Ho RC, McIntyre RS: Drug-drug interactions as a result of co-administering Δ9-THC and CBD with other psychotropic agents. Expert Opin Drug Saf. 2018 Jan;17(1):51-54. doi: 10.1080/14740338.2017.1397128.

[618] Monographie NN. Cannabidiol. Deutscher Arzneimittel-Codex (DAC) inkl. Neues Rezeptur-Formularium (NRF). DAC/NRF October 22, 2015.

[619] Brzozowska N, Li KM, Wang XS, Booth J, Stuart J, McGregor IS, Arnold JC: ABC transporters P-gp and Bcrp do not limit the brain uptake of the novel antipsychotic and anticonvulsant drug cannabidiol in mice. PeerJ. 2016 May 26;4:e2081. doi: 10.7717/peerj.2081.

[620] Grotenhermen F, Müller-Vahl K. Cannabis und Cannabinoide in der Medizin: Fakten und Ausblick. Suchttherapie. 2016;17:71–76.

[621] Corroon J, Phillips JA. A Cross-Sectional Study of Cannabidiol Users. Cannabis Cannabinoid Res. 2018;3(1):152–161. Published 2018 Jul 1. doi:10.1089/can.2018.0006.

[622] Gallily R, Yekhtin Z, Hanus LO: Overcoming the Bell-Shaped Dose-Response of Cannabidiol by Using Cannabis Extract Enriched in Cannabidiol. Pharmacology & Pharmacy, 2015, 6, 75-85. dx.doi.org/10.4236/pp.2015.62010.

[623] Corroon J, Phillips JA. A Cross-Sectional Study of Cannabidiol Users. Cannabis Cannabinoid Res. 2018;3(1):152–161. Published 2018 Jul 1. doi:10.1089/can.2018.0006.

[624] Bonn-Miller MO, Loflin MJE, Thomas BF, Marcu JP, Hyke T, Vandrey R: Labeling Accuracy of Cannabidiol Extracts Sold Online. JAMA. 2017 Nov 7;318(17):1708-1709. doi: 10.1001/jama.2017.11909.

[625] Mechoulam R, Hanus L: A historical overview of chemical research on cannabinoids. Chem Phys Lipids. 2000 Nov; 108(1-2):1-13. PMID: 11106779.

[626] Gertsch J, Pertwee RG, Di Marzo V: Phytocannabinoids beyond the Cannabis plant - do they exist? Br J Pharmacol. 2010;160(3):523-9. doi: 10.1111/j.1476-5381.2010.00745.x.

[627] Fellermeier M, Eisenreich W, Bacher A, Zenk MH: Biosynthesis of cannabinoids. Incorporation experiments with (13)C-labeled glucoses. Eur J Biochem. 2001 Mar;268(6):1596-604. PMID: 11248677.

[628] Russo EB. Taming THC: potential cannabis synergy and phytocannabinoid-terpenoid entourage effects. Br J Pharmacol. 2011;163(7):1344-64. doi: 10.1111/j.1476-5381.2011.01238.x.

[629] Giese MW, Lewis MA, Giese L, Smith KM: Development and Validation of a Reliable and Robust Method for the Analysis of Cannabinoids and Terpenes in

Cannabis. J AOAC Int. 2015 Nov-Dec;98(6):1503-22. doi: 10.5740/jaoacint.15-116.

[630] Pamplona FA, da Silva LR, Coan AC: Potential Clinical Benefits of CBD-Rich Cannabis Extracts Over Purified CBD in Treatment-Resistant Epilepsy: Observational Data Meta-analysis. Front Neurol. 2018;9:759. doi:10.3389/fneur.2018.00759.

[631] Kamal BS, Kamal F, Lantela DE: Cannabis and the Anxiety of Fragmentation-A Systems Approach for Finding an Anxiolytic Cannabis Chemotype. Front Neurosci. 2018;12:730. doi:10.3389/fnins.2018.00730.

[632] Gallily R, Yekhtin Z, Hanuš LO: Overcoming the Bell-Shaped Dose-Response of Cannabidiol by Using Cannabis Extract Enriched in Cannabidiol. Pharmacology & Pharmacy. Vol.6 No.2(2015), 75-85. doi:10.4236/pp.2015.62010.

[633] McPartland JM, Guy GW, Di Marzo V. Care and feeding of the endocannabinoid system: a systematic review of potential clinical interventions that upregulate the endocannabinoid system. PLoS One. 2014;9(3):e89566.. doi:10.1371/journal.pone.0089566.

[634] Kulig K: Interpretation of Workplace Tests for Cannabinoids. J Med Toxicol. 2016;13(1):106-110. doi: 10.1007/s13181-016-0587-z.

[635] Insurance Institute for Highway Safety (IIHS) and Highway Loss Data Institute (HLDI). Crashes rise in first states to begin legalized retail sales of recreational marijuana. iihs.org/iihs/news/desktopnews/crashes-rise-in-first-states-to-begin-legalized-retail-sales-of-recreational-marijuana.

[636] Nahler G, Grotenhermen F, Zuardi AW, Crippa JAS: A Conversion of Oral Cannabidiol to Delta9-Tetrahydrocannabinol Seems Not to Occur in Humans. Cannabis Cannabinoid Res. 2017;2(1):81-86. doi:10.1089/can.2017.0009.

[637] Bonn-Miller MO, Loflin MJE, Thomas BF, Marcu JP, Hyke T, Vandrey R. Labeling Accuracy of Cannabidiol Extracts Sold Online. JAMA. 2017;318(17):1708-1709. doi: 10.1001/jama.2017.11909.

[638] The U.S. Food and Drug Administration FDA: Scientific Data and Information about Products Containing Cannabis or Cannabis-Derived Compounds; Public Hearing. May 2019. www.fda.gov/news-events/fda-meetings-conferences-and-workshops/scientific-data-and-information-about-products-containing-cannabis-or-cannabis-derived-compounds.

[639] Taylor L, Gidal B, Blakey G, Tayo B, Morrison G: A Phase I, Randomized, Double-Blind, Placebo-Controlled, Single Ascending Dose, Multiple Dose, and Food Effect Trial of the Safety, Tolerability and Pharmacokinetics of Highly Purified Cannabidiol in Healthy Subjects. CNS Drugs. 2018 Nov;32(11):1053-1067. doi: 10.1007/s40263-018-0578-5.

[640] Toutain PL, Bousquet-Mélou A: Plasma terminal half-life. J Vet Pharmacol Ther. 2004 Dec;27(6):427-39. doi: 10.1111/j.1365-2885.2004.00600.x.

[641] Bergamaschi MM, Queiroz RH, Zuardi AW, Crippa JA: Safety and side effects of cannabidiol, a Cannabis sativa constituent. Curr Drug Saf. 2011 Sep 1;6(4):237-49. PMID: 22129319.

[642] Consroe P, Laguna J, Allender J, Snider S, Stern L, Sandyk R, Kennedy K, Schram K: Controlled clinical trial of cannabidiol in Huntington's disease. Pharmacol Biochem Behav. 1991 Nov;40(3):701-8. PMID: 1839644.

[643] Manini AF, Yiannoulos G, Bergamaschi MM, Hernandez S, Olmedo R, Barnes AJ, Winkel G, Sinha R, Jutras-Aswad D, Huestis MA, Hurd YL: Safety and pharmacokinetics of oral cannabidiol when administered concomitantly with intravenous fentanyl in humans. J Addict Med. 2015 May-Jun;9(3):204-10. doi: 10.1097/ADM.0000000000000118.

[644] Harvey DJ, Mechoulam R: Metabolites of cannabidiol identified in human urine. Xenobiotica. 1990 Mar;20(3):303-20. doi: 10.3109/00498259009046849.

[645] Bhattacharyya S, Morrison PD, Fusar-Poli P, et al. Opposite effects of delta-9-tetrahydrocannabinol and cannabidiol on human brain function and psychopathology. Neuropsychopharmacology. 2009;35(3):764–774. doi:10.1038/npp.2009.184.

[646] Martin-Santos R1, Crippa JA, Batalla A, Bhattacharyya S, Atakan Z, Borgwardt S, Allen P, Seal M, Langohr K, Farré M, Zuardi AW, McGuire PK: Acute effects of a single, oral dose of d9-tetrahydrocannabinol (THC) and cannabidiol (CBD) administration in healthy volunteers. Curr Pharm Des. 2012;18(32):4966-79. www.ncbi.nlm.nih.gov/pubmed/22716148.

[647] Crippa JA, Hallak JE, Machado-de-Sousa JP, Queiroz RH, Bergamaschi M, Chagas MH, Zuardi AW: Cannabidiol for the treatment of cannabis withdrawal syndrome: a case report. J Clin Pharm Ther. 2013 Apr;38(2): 162-4. doi: 10.1111/jcpt.12018.

[648] Devinsky O, Patel AD, Cross JH, Villanueva V, Wirrell EC, Privitera M, Greenwood SM, Roberts C, Checketts D, VanLandingham KE, Zuberi SM; GWPCARE Study Group: Effect of Cannabidiol on Drop Seizures in the Lennox-Gastaut Syndrome. N Engl J Med. 2018 May 17;378(20):1888-1897. doi: 10.1056/NEJMoa1714631.

[649] Thiele EA, Marsh ED, French JA, Mazurkiewicz-Beldzinska M, Benbadis SR, Joshi C, Lyons PD, Taylor A, Roberts C, Sommerville K; GWPCARE4 Study Group: Cannabidiol in patients with seizures associated with Lennox-Gastaut syndrome (GWPCARE4): a randomised, double-blind, placebo-controlled phase 3 trial. Lancet. 2018 Mar 17;391(10125):1085-1096. doi: 10.1016/S0140-6736(18)30136-3.

[650] Bergamaschi MM, Queiroz RH, Chagas MH, de Oliveira DC, De Martinis BS, Kapczinski F, Quevedo J, Roesler R, Schröder N, Nardi AE, Martín-Santos R, Hallak JE, Zuardi AW, Crippa JA: Cannabidiol reduces the anxiety induced by simulated public speaking in treatment-naïve social phobia patients. Neuropsychopharmacology. 2011 May;36(6):1219-26. doi: 10.1038/npp.2011.6.

[651] Perucca E. Cannabinoids in the Treatment of Epilepsy: Hard Evidence at Last?. J Epilepsy Res. 2017;7(2):61–76. doi:10.14581/jer.17012.

[652] Kogan L, Schoenfeld-Tacher R, Hellyer P, Rishniw M: US Veterinarians' Knowledge, Experience, and Perception Regarding the Use of Cannabidiol for Canine Medical Conditions. Front Vet Sci. 2019 Jan 10;5:338. doi: 10.3389/fvets.2018.00338.

[653] Gamble LJ, Boesch JM, Frye CW, et al. Pharmacokinetics, Safety, and Clinical Efficacy of Cannabidiol Treatment in Osteoarthritic Dogs. Front Vet Sci. 2018;5:165. Published 2018 Jul 23. doi:10.3389/fvets.2018.00165.

[654] Samara E, Bialer M, Mechoulam R: Pharmacokinetics of cannabidiol in dogs. Drug Metab Dispos. 1988 May-Jun;16(3):469-72. PMID: 2900742.

[655] Petty M: DVM360 Magazine. Cannabidiol: A new option for pets in pain? veterinarynews.dvm360.com/cannabidiol-new-option-pets-pain.

[656] Guiden M: Preliminary data from CBD clinical trials 'promising' News From The College Of Veterinary Medicine And Biomedical Sciences, Colorado State University. cvmbs.source.colostate.edu/preliminary-data-from-cbd-clinical-trials-promising.

[657] American Kennel Club Canine Health Foundation. Can CBD Oil Help Dogs With Epilepsy? The AKC Canine Health Foundation Investigates. 2018. www.akc.org/expert-advice/health/cbd-oil-for-dog-seizures.

[658] Dwyer JD: The central American, west Indian, and South American species of copaifera (caesalpiniaceae). Brittonia (1951) 7: 143. doi.org/10.2307/2804703.

[659] Plants For A Future: Copaifera officinalis - L. pfaf.org/user/Plant.aspx?LatinName=Copaifera+officinalis.

[660] Da Trindade R, Kelly da Silva J, William N. Setzer: Copaifera of the Neotropics: A Review of the Phytochemistry and Pharmacology. Int. J. Mol. Sci. 2018, 19(5), 1511; doi:10.3390/ijms19051511.

[661] Science Daily: Copaiba: Silver bullet or snake oil? www.sciencedaily.com/releases/2017/06/170606101417.htm.

[662] Veiga Junior VF, Rosas EC, Carvalho MV, Henriques MG, Pinto AC: Chemical composition and anti-inflammatory activity of copaiba oils from Copaifera cearensis Huber ex Ducke, Copaifera reticulata Ducke and Copaifera multijuga Hayne--a comparative study. J Ethnopharmacol. 2007 Jun 13;112(2):248-54. doi: 10.1016/j.jep.2007.03.005.

[663] Hendriks H, Malingre T, Battermann S, Boss R. Mono- and sesquiterpene hydrocarbons of the essential oil of Cannabis sativa. Phytochemistry. 1975;14:814–815.

[664] PubChem. Open Chemistry Database. Caryophyllene. National Institute of Health NIH, National Center for Biotechnology Information: pubchem.ncbi.nlm.nih.gov/compound/beta-caryophyllene.

[665] Orav A, Stulova I, Kailas T, Müürisepp M: Effect of storage on the essential oil composition of Piper nigrum L. fruits of different ripening states. J Agric Food Chem. 2004 May 5;52(9):2582-6. doi: 10.1021/jf030635s.

[666] Mockute D, Bernotiene G, Judzentiene A: The essential oil of Origanum vulgare L. ssp. vulgare growing wild in vilnius district (Lithuania). Phytochemistry. 2001 May;57(1):65-9. PMID: 11336262.

[667] Stewart D: The Chemistry of Essential Oils Made Simple. Chemical Analysis of Piper Nigrum. Care Publications 2013. Table 32. Pp 506-557.

[668] Gertsch J, Leonti M, Raduner S, et al: Beta-caryophyllene is a dietary cannabinoid. Proc Natl Acad Sci U S A. 2008;105(26):9099-104. doi: 10.1073/pnas.0803601105.

[669] Gertsch J, Leonti M, Raduner S, Racz I, Chen JZ, Xie XQ, Altmann KH, Karsak M, Zimmer A: Beta-caryophyllene is a dietary cannabinoid. Proc Natl Acad Sci U S A. 2008 Jul 1;105(26):9099-104. doi: 10.1073/pnas.0803601105.

[670] Zimmer A, Racz I, Klauke AL, Markert A, Gertsch J: Beta-caryophyllene, a phytocannabinoid acting on CB2 receptors. 2009. IACM 5th Conference on cannabinoids in medicine, 2-3.Oct, Cologne, Germany.

[671] Klauke AL, Racz I, Pradier B, Markert A, Zimmer AM, Gertsch J, Zimmer A: The cannabinoid CB_2 receptor-selective phytocannabinoid beta-caryophyllene exerts analgesic effects in mouse models of inflammatory and neuropathic pain. Eur Neuropsychopharmacol. 2014 Apr;24(4):608-20. doi: 10.1016/j.euroneuro.2013.10.008.

[672] Viveros-Paredes JM, González-Castañeda RE, Gertsch J, et al: Neuroprotective Effects of β-Caryophyllene against Dopaminergic Neuron Injury in a Murine Model of Parkinson's Disease Induced by MPTP. Pharmaceuticals (Basel). 2017;10(3):60. Published 2017 Jul 6. doi:10.3390/ph10030060.

[673] Ames-Sibin AP, Barizão CL, Castro-Ghizoni CV, Silva FMS, Sá-Nakanishi AB, Bracht L, Bersani-Amado CA, Marçal-Natali MR, Bracht A, Comar JF: β-Caryophyllene, the major constituent of copaiba oil, reduces systemic inflammation and oxidative stress in arthritic rats. J Cell Biochem. 2018 Dec;119(12):10262-10277. doi: 10.1002/jcb.27369.

[674] Fidyt K, Fiedorowicz A, Strządała L, Szumny A: β-caryophyllene and β-caryophyllene oxide-natural compounds of anticancer and analgesic properties. Cancer Med. 2016;5(10):3007-3017. doi: 10.1002/cam4.816

[675] Teixeira FB, de Brito Silva R, Lameira OA, Webber LP, D'Almeida Couto RS, Martins MD, Lima RR: Copaiba oil-resin (Copaifera reticulata Ducke) modulates the inflammation in a model of injury to rats' tongues. BMC Complement Altern Med. 2017 Jun 14;17(1):313. doi: 10.1186/s12906-017-1820-2.

[676] Guimarães-Santos A, Santos DS, Santos IR, et al. Copaiba oil-resin treatment is neuroprotective and reduces neutrophil recruitment and microglia activation after motor cortex excitotoxic injury. Evid Based Complement Alternat Med. 2012;2012:918174. doi: 10.1155/2012/918174.

[677] Curio M, Jacone H, Perrut J, Pinto AC, Filho VF, Silva RC: Acute effect of Copaifera reticulata Ducke copaiba oil in rats tested in the elevated plus-maze: an ethological analysis. J Pharm Pharmacol. 2009 Aug;61(8):1105-10. doi: 10.1211/jpp.61.08.0015.

[678] Castro Ghizoni CV, Arssufi Ames AP, Lameira OA, Bersani Amado CA, Sá Nakanishi AB, Bracht 1, Marçal Natali MR, Peralta RM, Bracht A, Comar JF: Anti-Inflammatory and Antioxidant Actions of Copaiba Oil Are Related to Liver Cell Modifications in Arthritic Rats. J Cell Biochem. 2017 Oct;118(10):3409-3423. doi: 10.1002/jcb.25998.

[679] Bahr T, Allred K, Martinez D, Rodriguez D, Winterton P: Effects of a massage-like essential oil application procedure using Copaiba and Deep Blue oils in individuals with hand arthritis. Complement Ther Clin Pract. 2018 Nov;33:170-176. doi: 10.1016/j.ctcp.2018.10.004.

[680] Koulivand PH, Khaleghi Ghadiri M, Gorji A. Lavender and the nervous system. Evid Based Complement Alternat Med. 2013;2013:681304. doi: 10.1155/2013/681304.

[681] Keshavarz Afshar M, Behboodi Moghadam Z, Taghizadeh Z, Bekhradi R, Montazeri A, Mokhtari P. Lavender fragrance essential oil and the quality of

sleep in postpartum women. Iran Red Crescent Med J. 2015;17(4):e25880. doi:10.5812/ircmj.17(4)2015.25880.

[682] Chen SL, Chen CH: Effects of Lavender Tea on Fatigue, Depression, and Maternal-Infant Attachment in Sleep-Disturbed Postnatal Women. Worldviews Evid Based Nurs. 2015 Dec;12(6):370-9. doi: 10.1111/wvn.12122.

[683] Lillehei AS, Halcón LL, Savik K, Reis R. Effect of Inhaled Lavender and Sleep Hygiene on Self-Reported Sleep Issues: A Randomized Controlled Trial. J Altern Complement Med. 2015;21(7):430-8. doi: 10.1089/acm.2014.0327.

[684] Lee IS, Lee GJ: Effects of lavender aromatherapy on insomnia and depression in women college students. Taehan Kanho Hakhoe Chi. 2006 Feb;36(1):136-43. PMID: 16520572.

[685] Ozkaraman A, Dügüm Ö, Özen Yılmaz H, Usta Yesilbalkan Ö: Aromatherapy: The Effect of Lavender on Anxiety and Sleep Quality in Patients Treated With Chemotherapy. Clin J Oncol Nurs. 2018 Apr 1;22(2):203-210. doi: 10.1188/18.CJON.203-210.

[686] Şentürk A, Tekinsoy Kartın P: The Effect of Lavender Oil Application via Inhalation Pathway on Hemodialysis Patients' Anxiety Level and Sleep Quality. Holist Nurs Pract. 2018 Nov/Dec;32(6):324-335. doi: 10.1097/HNP.0000000000000292.

[687] López V, Nielsen B, Solas M, Ramírez MJ, Jäger AK. Exploring Pharmacological Mechanisms of Lavender (Lavandula angustifolia) Essential Oil on Central Nervous System Targets. Front Pharmacol. 2017;8:280. doi:10.3389/fphar.2017.00280.

[688] Malcolm BJ, Tallian K. Essential oil of lavender in anxiety disorders: Ready for prime time?. Ment Health Clin. 2018;7(4):147-155. doi:10.9740/mhc.2017.07.147.

[689] Schuwald AM, Nöldner M, Wilmes T, Klugbauer N, Leuner K, Müller WE: Lavender oil-potent anxiolytic properties via modulating voltage dependent calcium channels. PLoS One. 2013 Apr 29;8(4):e59998. doi: 10.1371/journal.pone.0059998.

[690] Global Online Essential Oils Symposiums 2017, 2018, and 2019. www.DoctorOli.com.

[691] Lee BH, Lee JS, Kim YC. Hair Growth-Promoting Effects of Lavender Oil in C57BL/6 Mice. Toxicol Res. 2016;32(2):103-8. doi: 10.5487/TR.2016.32.2.103

[692] Sasannejad P, Saeedi M, Shoeibi A, Gorji A, Abbasi M, Foroughipour M: Lavender essential oil in the treatment of migraine headache: a placebo-controlled clinical trial. Eur Neurol. 2012;67(5):288-91. doi: 10.1159/000335249. Epub 2012 Apr 17.

[693] Nasiri A, Mahmodi MA, Nobakht Z: Effect of aromatherapy massage with lavender essential oil on pain in patients with osteoarthritis of the knee: A randomized controlled clinical trial. Complement Ther Clin Pract. 2016 Nov;25:75-80. doi: 10.1016/j.ctcp.2016.08.002

[694] Nasiri A, Mahmodi MA: Aromatherapy massage with lavender essential oil and the prevention of disability in ADL in patients with osteoarthritis of the knee: A randomized controlled clinical trial. Complement Ther Clin Pract. 2018 Feb;30:116-121. doi: 10.1016/j.ctcp.2017.12.012.

[695] Woollard AC, Tatham KC, Barker S: The influence of essential oils on the process of wound healing: a review of the current evidence. J Wound Care. 2007 Jun;16(6):255-7. doi: 10.12968/jowc.2007.16.6.27064.

[696] Altaei DT: Topical lavender oil for the treatment of recurrent aphthous ulceration. Am J Dent. 2012 Feb;25(1):39-43. PMID: 22558691.

[697] Mori HM, Kawanami H, Kawahata H, Aoki M: Wound healing potential of lavender oil by acceleration of granulation and wound contraction through induction of TGF-β in a rat model. BMC Complement Altern Med. 2016 May 26;16:144. doi: 10.1186/s12906-016-1128-7.

[698] Sheikhan F, Jahdi F, Khoei EM, Shamsalizadeh N, Sheikhan M, Haghani H: Episiotomy pain relief: Use of Lavender oil essence in primiparous Iranian women. Complement Ther Clin Pract. 2012 Feb;18(1):66-70. doi: 10.1016/j.ctcp.2011.02.003.

[699] Nikjou R, Kazemzadeh R, Rostamnegad M, Moshfegi S, Karimollahi M, Salehi H: The Effect of Lavender Aromatherapy on the Pain Severity of Primary Dysmenorrhea: A Triple-blind Randomized Clinical Tserial. Ann Med Health Sci Res. 2016 Jul-Aug;6(4):211-215. doi: 10.4103/amhsr.amhsr_527_14.

[700] National Center for Complementary and Integrative Health. Peppermint Oil. nccih.nih.gov/health/peppermintoil.

[701] Meamarbashi A. Instant effects of peppermint essential oil on the physiological parameters and exercise performance. Avicenna J Phytomed. 2014;4(1):72-8. PMID: 25050303.

[702] Meamarbashi A, Rajabi A. The effects of peppermint on exercise performance. J Int Soc Sports Nutr. 2013;10(1):15. Published 2013 Mar 21. doi:10.1186/1550-2783-10-15.

[703] Thompson AJ, Lummis SC. 5-HT3 receptors. Curr Pharm Des. 2006;12(28):3615-30. PMID: 17073663.

[704] Ashoor A, Nordman JC, Veltri D, Yang KH, Shuba Y, Al Kury L, Sadek B, Howarth FC, Shehu A, Kabbani N, Oz M: Menthol inhibits 5-HT3 receptor-mediated currents. J Pharmacol Exp Ther. 2013 Nov;347(2): 398-409. doi: 10.1124/jpet.113.203976.

[705] Yang KH, Galadari S, Isaev D, Petroianu G, Shippenberg TS, Oz M: The nonpsychoactive cannabinoid cannabidiol inhibits 5-hydroxytryptamine3A receptor-mediated currents in Xenopus laevis oocytes. J Pharmacol Exp Ther. 2010 May;333(2):547-54. doi: 10.1124/jpet.109.162594.

[706] Oz M, Zhang L, Morales M: Endogenous cannabinoid, anandamide, acts as a noncompetitive inhibitor on 5-HT3 receptor-mediated responses in Xenopus oocytes. Synapse. 2002 Dec 1;46(3):150-6. doi: 10.1002/syn.10121.

[707] Lane B, Cannella K, Bowen C, Copelan D, Nteff G, Barnes K, Poudevigne M, Lawson J: Examination of the effectiveness of peppermint aromatherapy on nausea in women post C-section. J Holist Nurs. 2012 Jun;30(2):90-104; quiz 105-6. doi: 10.1177/0898010111423419.

[708] Briggs P, Hawrylack H, Mooney R: Inhaled peppermint oil for postop nausea in patients undergoing cardiac surgery. Nursing. 2016 Jul;46(7):61-7. doi: 10.1097/01.NURSE.0000482882.38607.5c.

[709] Pasha H, Behmanesh F, Mohsenzadeh F, Hajahmadi M, Moghadamnia AA: Study of the effect of mint oil on nausea and vomiting during pregnancy. Iran Red Crescent Med J. 2012 Nov;14(11):727-30. doi: 10.5812/ircmj.3477.

[710] Joulaeerad N, Ozgoli G, Hajimehdipoor H, Ghasemi E, Salehimoghaddam F: Effect of Aromatherapy with Peppermint Oil on the Severity of Nausea and Vomiting in Pregnancy: A Single-blind, Randomized, Placebo-controlled trial. J Reprod Infertil. 2018 Jan-Mar;19(1):32-38. PMID: 29850445.

[711] Tate S: Peppermint oil: a treatment for postoperative nausea. J Adv Nurs. 1997 Sep;26(3):543-9. PMID: 9378876.

[712] Lua PL, Zakaria NS: A brief review of current scientific evidence involving aromatherapy use for nausea and vomiting. J Altern Complement Med. 2012 Jun;18(6):534-40. doi: 10.1089/acm.2010.0862.

[713] Oh JY, Park MA, Kim YC. Peppermint Oil Promotes Hair Growth without Toxic Signs. Toxicol Res. 2014;30(4):297-304: doi: 10.5487/TR.2014.30.4.297.

[714] Hay IC, Jamieson M, Ormerod AD: Randomized trial of aromatherapy. Successful treatment for alopecia areata. Arch Dermatol. 1998 Nov;134(11):1349-52. PMID: 9828867.

[715] Moss M, Hewitt S, Moss L, Wesnes K: Modulation of cognitive performance and mood by aromas of peppermint and ylang-ylang. Int J Neurosci. 2008 Jan;118(1):59-77. doi: 10.1080/00207450601042094.

[716] Norrish MI, Dwyer KL: Preliminary investigation of the effect of peppermint oil on an objective measure of daytime sleepiness. Int J Psychophysiol. 2005 Mar;55(3):291-8. doi: 10.1016/j.ijpsycho.2004.08.004.

[717] Ho C, Spence C: Olfactory facilitation of dual-task performance. Neurosci Lett. 2005 Nov 25;389(1):35-40. doi: 10.1016/j.neulet.2005.07.003.

[718] Raudenbush B, Grayhem R, Sears T, Wilson I. Effects of peppermint and cinnamon odor administration on simulated driving alertness, mood and workload. N. Am. J. Psychol. 2009;11:245–256.

[719] Steward D; The Chemistry of Essential Oils. Care Publications 2013, 4th edition: Mentha piperita. Pg 537-538.

[720] McKemy DD: How cold is it? TRPM8 and TRPA1 in the molecular logic of cold sensation. Mol Pain. 2005 Apr 22;1:16. doi: 10.1186/1744-8069-1-16.

[721] De Petrocellis L, Ligresti A, Moriello AS, et al. Effects of cannabinoids and cannabinoid-enriched Cannabis extracts on TRP channels and endocannabinoid metabolic enzymes. Br J Pharmacol. 2011;163(7):1479-94. doi: 10.1111/j.1476-5381.2010.01166.x.

[722] De Petrocellis L, Vellani V, Schiano-Moriello A, Marini P, Magherini PC, Orlando P, Di Marzo V: Plant-derived cannabinoids modulate the activity of transient receptor potential channels of ankyrin type-1 and melastatin type-8. J Pharmacol Exp Ther. 2008 Jun;325(3):1007-15. doi: 10.1124/jpet.107.134809.

[723] Moussaieff A, Mechoulam R: Boswellia resin: from religious ceremonies to medical uses; a review of in-vitro, in-vivo and clinical trials. J Pharm Pharmacol. 2009 Oct;61(10):1281-93. doi: 10.1211/jpp/61.10.0003.

[724] Chevrier MR, Ryan AE, Lee DY, Zhongze M, Wu-Yan Z, Via CS: Boswellia carterii extract inhibits TH1 cytokines and promotes TH2 cytokines in vitro. Clin Diagn Lab Immunol. 2005 May;12(5):575-80. doi: 10.1128/CDLI.12.5.575-580.2005.

[725] Akihisa T, Tabata K, Banno N, Tokuda H, Nishimura R, Nakamura Y, Kimura Y, Yasukawa K, Suzuki T: Cancer chemopreventive effects and cytotoxic activities of the triterpene acids from the resin of Boswellia carteri. Biol Pharm Bull. 2006 Sep;29(9):1976-9. PMID: 16946522.

[726] Al-Yasiry AR, Kiczorowska B: Frankincense-therapeutic properties. Postepy Hig Med Dosw (Online).2016 Jan 4;70:380-91.PMID:27117114.

[727] Banno N, Akihisa T, Yasukawa K, Tokuda H, Tabata K, Nakamura Y, Nishimura R, Kimura Y, Suzuki T: Anti-inflammatory activities of the triterpene acids from the resin of Boswellia carteri. J Ethnopharmacol. 2006 Sep 19;107(2):249-53. doi: 10.1016/j.jep.2006.03.006.

[728] Li XJ, Yang YJ, Li YS, Zhang WK, Tang HB: α-Pinene, linalool, and 1-octanol contribute to the topical anti-inflammatory and analgesic activities of frankincense by inhibiting COX-2. J Ethnopharmacol. 2016 Feb 17;179:22-6. doi: 10.1016/j.jep.2015.12.039.

[729] Su S, Hua Y, Wang Y, Gu W, Zhou W, Duan JA, Jiang H, Chen T, Tang Y: Evaluation of the anti-inflammatory and analgesic properties of individual and combined extracts from Commiphora myrrha, and Boswellia carterii. J Ethnopharmacol. 2012 Jan 31;139(2):649-56. doi: 10.1016/j.jep.2011.12.013.

[730] A randomized, double blind, placebo controlled, cross over study to evaluate the analgesic activity of Boswellia serrata in healthy volunteers using mechanical pain model. Indian J Pharmacol. 2014;46(5):475-9. doi: 10.4103/0253-7613.140570.

[731] Kimmatkar N, Thawani V, Hingorani L, Khiyani R: Efficacy and tolerability of Boswellia serrata extract in treatment of osteoarthritis of knee--a randomized double blind placebo controlled trial. Phytomedicine. 2003 Jan;10(1):3-7. doi: 10.1078/094471103321648593.

[732] Abdel-Tawab M, Werz O, Schubert-Zsilavecz M: Boswellia serrata: an overall assessment of in vitro, preclinical, pharmacokinetic and clinical data. Clin Pharmacokinet. 2011 Jun;50(6):349-69. doi: 10.2165/11586800-000000000-00000.

[733] Long-term efficacy of Boswellia serrata in 4 patients with chronic cluster headache. J Headache Pain. 2013;14(Suppl 1):P37. doi: 10.1186/1129-2377-14-S1-P37.

[734] Moussaieff A, Rimmerman N, Bregman T, et al. Incensole acetate, an incense component, elicits psychoactivity by activating TRPV3 channels in the brain. FASEB J. 2008;22(8):3024-34. doi: 10.1096/fj.07-101865.

[735] Moussaieff A, Gross M, Nesher E, Tikhonov T, Yadid G, Pinhasov A: Incensole acetate reduces depressive-like behavior and modulates hippocampal BDNF and CRF expression of submissive animals. J Psychopharmacol. 2012 Dec;26(12):1584-93. doi: 10.1177/0269881112458729.

[736] Science Direct: Burning Incense Is Psychoactive: New Class Of Antidepressants Might Be Right Under Our Noses. www.sciencedaily.com/releases/2008/05/080520110415.htm.

[737] Suhail MM, Wu W, Cao A, Mondalek FG, Fung KM, Shih PT, Fang YT, Woolley C, Young G, Lin HK: Boswellia sacra essential oil induces tumor cell-specific apoptosis and suppresses tumor aggressiveness in cultured human

breast cancer cells. BMC Complement Altern Med. 2011 Dec 15;11:129. doi: 10.1186/1472-6882-11-129.

[738] Shao Y, Ho CT, Chin CK, Badmaev V, Ma W, Huang MT: Inhibitory activity of boswellic acids from Boswellia serrata against human leukemia HL-60 cells in culture. Planta Med. 1998 May;64(4):328-31. doi: 10.1055/s-2006-957444.

[739] Xia D, Lou W, Fung KM, Wolley CL, Suhail MM, Lin HK. Cancer Chemopreventive Effects of Boswellia sacra Gum Resin Hydrodistillates on Invasive Urothelial Cell Carcinoma: Report of a Case. Integr Cancer Ther. 2016;16(4):605-611. doi: 10.1177/1534735416664174.

[740] Winking M, Sarikaya S, Rahmanian A, Jödicke A, Böker DK: Boswellic acids inhibit glioma growth: a new treatment option? J Neurooncol. 2000;46(2):97-103. PMID: 10894362.

[741] Flavin DF: A lipoxygenase inhibitor in breast cancer brain metastases. J Neurooncol. 2007 Mar;82(1):91-3. doi: 10.1007/s11060-006-9248-4.

[742] Conti S, Vexler A, Edry-Botzer L, Kalich-Philosoph L, Corn BW, Shtraus N, Meir Y, Hagoel L, Shtabsky A, Marmor S, Earon G, Lev-Ari S: Combined acetyl-11-keto-β-boswellic acid and radiation treatment inhibited glioblastoma tumor cells. PLoS One. 2018 Jul 3;13(7):e0198627. doi: 10.1371/journal.pone.0198627.

[743] Hostanska K, Daum G, Saller R: Cytostatic and apoptosis-inducing activity of boswellic acids toward malignant cell lines in vitro. Anticancer Res. 2002 Sep-Oct;22(5):2853-62. PMID: 12530009.

[744] Dosoky NS, Setzer WN. Biological Activities and Safety of Citrus spp. Essential Oils. Int J Mol Sci. 2018;19(7):1966. doi:10.3390/ijms19071966.

[745] Ibrahim EA, Wang M, Radwan MM, Wanas AS, Majumdar CG, Avula B, Wang YH, Khan IA, Chandra S, Lata H, Hadad GM, Abdel Salam RA, Ibrahim AK, Ahmed SA, ElSohly MA: Analysis of Terpenes in Cannabis sativa L. Using GC/MS: Method Development, Validation, and Application. Planta Med. 2019 Mar;85(5):431-438. doi: 10.1055/a-0828-8387.

[746] Marshall JR: Improving Americans' diet--setting public policy with limited knowledge. Am J Public Health. 1995 Dec;85(12):1609-11. PMID: 7503329.

[747] Tisserand R., Young R. Essential Oil Safety. 2nd ed. Elsevier; New York, NY, USA: 2014.

[748] Crowell PL, Gould MN: Chemoprevention and therapy of cancer by d-limonene. Crit Rev Oncog. 1994;5(1):1-22. PMID: 7948106.

[749] de Almeida AA, Costa JP, de Carvalho RB, de Sousa DP, de Freitas RM: Evaluation of acute toxicity of a natural compound (+)-limonene epoxide and its anxiolytic-like action. Brain Res. 2012 Apr 11;1448:56-62. doi: 10.1016/j.brainres.2012.01.070.

[750] Hirota R, Roger NN, Nakamura H, Song HS, Sawamura M, Suganuma N: Anti-inflammatory effects of limonene from yuzu (Citrus junos Tanaka) essential oil on eosinophils. J Food Sci. 2010 Apr;75(3):H87-92. doi: 10.1111/j.1750-3841.2010.01541.x.

[751] Cha JH, Lee SH, Yoo YS: Effects of aromatherapy on changes in the autonomic nervous system, aortic pulse wave velocity and aortic augmentation index in patients with essential hypertension. J Korean Acad Nurs. 2010 Oct;40(5):705-13. doi: 10.4040/jkan.2010.40.5.705.

[752] Lee H, Woo M, Kim M, Noh JS, Song YO. Antioxidative and Cholesterol-Lowering Effects of Lemon Essential Oil in Hypercholesterolemia-Induced Rabbits. Prev Nutr Food Sci. 2018;23(1):8-14. doi: 10.3746/pnf.2018.23.1.8.

[753] Komori T, Fujiwara R, Tanida M, Nomura J, Yokoyama MM: Effects of citrus fragrance on immune function and depressive states. Neuroimmunomodulation. 1995 May-Jun;2(3):174-80. doi: 10.1159/000096889.

[754] Zhou W, Yoshioka M, Yokogoshi H: Sub-chronic effects of s-limonene on brain neurotransmitter levels and behavior of rats. J Nutr Sci Vitaminol (Tokyo). 2009 Aug;55(4):367-73. PMID: 19763039.

[755] Yun J: Limonene inhibits methamphetamine-induced locomotor activity via regulation of 5-HT neuronal function and dopamine release. Phytomedicine. 2014 May 15;21(6):883-7. doi: 10.1016/j.phymed.2013.12.004.

[756] Costa CA, Cury TC, Cassettari BO, Takahira RK, Flório JC, Costa M. Citrus aurantium L. essential oil exhibits anxiolytic-like activity mediated by 5-HT(1A)-receptors and reduces cholesterol after repeated oral treatment. BMC Complement Altern Med. 2013;13:42. doi:10.1186/1472-6882-13-42.

[757] Hoenen M, Müller K, Pause BM, Lübke KT. Fancy Citrus, Feel Good: Positive Judgment of Citrus Odor, but Not the Odor Itself, Is Associated with Elevated Mood during Experienced Helplessness. Front Psychol. 2016;7:74. doi:10.3389/fpsyg.2016.00074.

[758] Lehrner J, Eckersberger C, Walla P, Pötsch G, Deecke L: Ambient odor of orange in a dental office reduces anxiety and improves mood in female patients. Physiol Behav. 2000 Oct 1-15;71(1-2):83-6. PMID: 11134689.

[759] Hasheminia D, Kalantar Motamedi MR, Karimi Ahmadabadi F, Hashemzehi H, Haghighat A: Can ambient orange fragrance reduce patient anxiety during surgical removal of impacted mandibular third molars? J Oral Maxillofac Surg. 2014 Sep;72(9):1671-6. doi: 10.1016/j.joms.2014.03.031.

[760] Wang X, Li G, Shen W. Protective effects of D-Limonene against transient cerebral ischemia in stroke-prone spontaneously hypertensive rats. Exp Ther Med. 2017;15(1):699-706. doi: 10.3892/etm.2017.5509.

[761] Wang L, Wang J, Fang L, et al. Anticancer activities of citrus peel polymethoxyflavones related to angiogenesis and others. Biomed Res Int. 2014;2014:453972. doi: 10.1155/2014/453972.

[762] Cirmi S, Maugeri A, Ferlazzo N, et al. Anticancer Potential of Citrus Juices and Their Extracts: A Systematic Review of Both Preclinical and Clinical Studies. Front Pharmacol. 2017;8:420. doi:10.3389/fphar.2017.00420.

[763] Cirmi S, Navarra M, Woodside JV, Cantwell MM: Citrus fruits intake and oral cancer risk: A systematic review and meta-analysis. Pharmacol Res. 2018 Jul;133:187-194. doi: 10.1016/j.phrs.2018.05.008.

[764] Song JK, Bae JM: Citrus fruit intake and breast cancer risk: a quantitative systematic review. J Breast Cancer. 2013 Mar;16(1):72-6. doi: 10.4048/jbc.2013.16.1.72.

[765] Bae JM, Lee EJ, Guyatt G: Citrus fruit intake and pancreatic cancer risk: a quantitative systematic review. Pancreas. 2009 Mar;38(2):168-74. doi: 10.1097/MPA.0b013e318188c497.

[766] Naganuma M, Hirose S, Nakayama Y, Nakajima K, Someya T: A study of the phototoxicity of lemon oil. Arch Dermatol Res. 1985;278(1):31-6. PMID: 4096528.

[767] Choi JY, Hwang S, Lee SH, Oh SH. Asymptomatic Hyperpigmentation without Preceding Inflammation as a Clinical Feature of Citrus Fruits-Induced Phytophotodermatitis. Ann Dermatol. 2017;30(1):75-78. doi: 10.5021/ad.2018.30.1.75.

[768] Weber IC, Davis CP, Greeson DM: Phytophotodermatitis: the other "lime" disease. J Emerg Med. 1999 Mar-Apr;17(2):235-7. PMID: 10195477.

[769] Wagner AM, Wu JJ, Hansen RC, Nigg HN, Beiere RC: Bullous phytophotodermatitis associated with high natural concentrations of furanocoumarins in limes. Am J Contact Dermat. 2002 Mar;13(1):10-4. PMID: 11887098.

[770] Khachemoune A, Khechmoune K, Blanc D: Assessing phytophotodermatitis: boy with erythema and blisters on both hands. Dermatol Nurs. 2006 Apr;18(2):153-4. PMID: 16708677.

[771] Ballabeni V, Tognolini M, Giorgio C, Bertoni S, Bruni R, Barocelli E: Ocotea quixos Lam. essential oil: in vitro and in vivo investigation on its anti-inflammatory properties. Fitoterapia. 2010 Jun;81(4):289-95. doi: 10.1016/j.fitote.2009.10.002.

[772] Ballabeni V, Tognolini M, Bertoni S, Bruni R, Guerrini A, Rueda GM, Barocelli E: Antiplatelet and antithrombotic activities of essential oil from wild Ocotea quixos (Lam.) Kosterm. (Lauraceae) calices from Amazonian Ecuador. Pharmacol Res. 2007 Jan;55(1):23-30. doi: 10.1016/j.phrs.2006.09.009.

[773] Ogundajo AL, Adeniran LA1, Ashafa AO: Medicinal properties of Ocotea bullata stem bark extracts: phytochemical constituents, antioxidant and anti-inflammatory activity, cytotoxicity and inhibition of carbohydrate-metabolizing enzymes. J Integr Med. 2018 Mar;16(2):132-140. doi: 10.1016/j.joim.2018.02.007.

[774] Babar A, Al-Wabel NA, Shams S, Aftab A, Khan SA, Anwar F: Essential oils used in aromatherapy: A systemic review. Asian Pacific Journal of Tropical Biomedicine. Volume 5, Issue 8, August 2015, Pages 601-611. doi.org/10.1016/j.apjtb.2015.05.007.

[775] Zhang N, Zhang L, Feng L, Yao L: The anxiolytic effect of essential oil of Cananga odorata exposure on mice and determination of its major active constituents. Phytomedicine. 2016 Dec 15;23(14):1727-1734. doi: 10.1016/j.phymed.2016.10.017.

[776] Zhang N, Zhang L, Feng L, Yao L: Cananga odorata essential oil reverses the anxiety induced by 1-(3-chlorophenyl) piperazine through regulating the MAPK pathway and serotonin system in mice. J Ethnopharmacol. 2018 Jun 12;219:23-30. doi: 10.1016/j.jep.2018.03.013.

[777] Hongratanaworakit T, Buchbauer G: Evaluation of the harmonizing effect of ylang-ylang oil on humans after inhalation. Planta Med. 2004 Jul;70(7):632-6. doi: 10.1055/s-2004-827186.

[778] Hongratanaworakit T, Buchbauer G: Relaxing effect of ylang ylang oil on humans after transdermal absorption. Phytother Res. 2006 Sep;20(9):758-63. doi: 10.1002/ptr.1950.

[779] Gnatta JR, Piason P, Lopes Cde L, Rogenski NM, Silva MJ: Aromatherapy with ylang ylang for anxiety and self-esteem: a pilot study. Rev Esc Enferm USP, 48 (3) (2014), pp. 492-499.

[780] Burdock GA, Carabin IG: Safety assessment of Ylang-Ylang (Cananga spp.) as a food ingredient. Food Chem Toxicol. 2008 Feb;46(2):433-45. doi: 10.1016/j.fct.2007.09.105.

[781] Elmhalli F, Pålsson K, Örberg J, Grandi G: Acaricidal properties of ylang-ylang oil and star anise oil against nymphs of Ixodes ricinus (Acari: Ixodidae). Exp Appl Acarol. 2018 Oct;76(2):209-220. doi: 10.1007/s10493-018-0299-y.

[782] Tan LT, Lee LH, Yin WF, et al. Traditional Uses, Phytochemistry, and Bioactivities of Cananga odorata (Ylang-Ylang). Evid Based Complement Alternat Med. 2015;2015:896314. doi: 10.1155/2015/896314.

[783] Steward D; The Chemistry of Essential Oils. Care Publications 2013, 4th edition: Canaga odorata. Pg 514-515.

[784] Singh G, Maurya S, DeLampasona MP, Catalan CA: A comparison of chemical, antioxidant and antimicrobial studies of cinnamon leaf and bark volatile oils, oleoresins and their constituents. Food Chem Toxicol. 2007 Sep;45(9):1650-61.

[785] Ranasinghe P, Pigera S, Premakumara GA, Galappaththy P, Constantine GR, Katulanda P: Medicinal properties of 'true' cinnamon (Cinnamomum zeylanicum): a systematic review. BMC Complement Altern Med. 2013 Oct 22;13:275. doi: 10.1186/1472-6882-13-275.

[786] Hariri M, Ghiasvand R: Cinnamon and Chronic Diseases. Adv Exp Med Biol. 2016;929:1-24.

[787] Yap PS, Krishnan T, Chan KG, Lim SH: Antibacterial Mode of Action of Cinnamomum verum Bark Essential Oil, Alone and in Combination with Piperacillin, Against a Multi-Drug-Resistant Escherichia coli Strain. J Microbiol Biotechnol. 2015 Aug;25(8):1299-306. doi: 10.4014/jmb.1407.07054.

[788] Ranasinghe P, Galappaththy P, Constantine GR, Jayawardena R, Weeratunga HD, Premakumara S, Katulanda P: Cinnamomum zeylanicum (Ceylon cinnamon) as a potential pharmaceutical agent for type-2 diabetes mellitus: study protocol for a randomized controlled trial. Trials. 2017 Sep 29;18(1):446. doi: 10.1186/s13063-017-2192-0.

[789] Jayaprakasha GK, Rao LJ: Chemistry, biogenesis, and biological activities of Cinnamomum zeylanicum. Crit Rev Food Sci Nutr. 2011 Jul;51(6):547-62. doi: 10.1080/10408391003699550.

[790] Dorri M, Hashemitabar S, Hosseinzadeh H: Cinnamon (Cinnamomum zeylanicum) as an antidote or a protective agent against natural or chemical toxicities: a review. Drug Chem Toxicol. 2018 Jul;41(3):338-351. doi: 10.1080/01480545.2017.1417995.

[791] Sangal A: Role of cinnamon as beneficial antidiabetic food adjunct: a review. Advances in Applied Science Research, 2011, 2 (4):440-450

[792] Mollazadeh H, Hosseinzadeh H. Cinnamon effects on metabolic syndrome: a review based on its mechanisms. Iran J Basic Med Sci. 2016;19(12):1258-1270. doi: 10.22038/ijbms.2016.7906.

[793] Anderson RA, Broadhurst CL, Polansky MM, Schmidt WF, Khan A, Flanagan VP, Schoene NW, Graves DJ: Isolation and characterization of

polyphenol type-A polymers from cinnamon with insulin-like biological activity. J Agric Food Chem. 2004 Jan 14;52(1):65-70. doi: 10.1021/jf034916b.

[794] Mang B, Wolters M, Schmitt B, Kelb K, Lichtinghagen R, Stichtenoth DO, Hahn A: Effects of a cinnamon extract on plasma glucose, HbA, and serum lipids in diabetes mellitus type 2. Eur J Clin Invest. 2006 May;36(5):340-4. doi: 10.1111/j.1365-2362.2006.01629.x.

[795] Khan A, Safdar M, Ali Khan MM, Khattak KN, Anderson RA: Cinnamon improves glucose and lipids of people with type 2 diabetes. Diabetes Care. 2003 Dec;26(12):3215-8. PMID: 14633804.

[796] Sengsuk C, Sanguanwong S, Tangvarasittichai O, Tangvarasittichai S: Effect of cinnamon supplementation on glucose, lipids levels, glomerular filtration rate, and blood pressure of subjects with type 2 diabetes mellitus. Diabetol Int. 2015 Jul 9;7(2):124-132. doi: 10.1007/s13340-015-0218-y..

[797] Maierean SM, Serban MC, Sahebkar A, Ursoniu S, Serban A, Penson P, Banach M; Lipid and Blood Pressure Meta-analysis Collaboration (LBPMC) Group: The effects of cinnamon supplementation on blood lipid concentrations: A systematic review and meta-analysis. J Clin Lipidol. 2017 Nov - Dec;11(6):1393-1406. doi: 10.1016/j.jacl.2017.08.004..

[798] Steward D; The Chemistry of Essential Oils. Care Publications 2013, 4th edition: Cinnamomum verum. Pg 518.

[799] Vigil JM, Stith SS, Diviant JP, Brockelman F, Keeling K, Hall B. Effectiveness of Raw, Natural Medical Cannabis Flower for Treating Insomnia under Naturalistic Conditions. Medicines (Basel). 2018;5(3):75. Published 2018 Jul 11. doi:10.3390/medicines5030075.

[800] Houghton PJ: The scientific basis for the reputed activity of Valerian. J Pharm Pharmacol. 1999 May;51(5):505-12. PMID: 10411208.

[801] Wang ZJ, Heinbockel T. Essential Oils and Their Constituents Targeting the GABAergic System and Sodium Channels as Treatment of Neurological Diseases. Molecules. 2018;23(5):1061. doi:10.3390/molecules23051061.

[802] Yuan CS, Mehendale S, Xiao Y, Aung HH, Xie JT, Ang-Lee MK: The gamma-aminobutyric acidergic effects of valerian and valerenic acid on rat brainstem neuronal activity. Anesth Analg. 2004 Feb;98(2):353-8. PMID: 14742369.

[803] Gottesmann C: GABA mechanisms and sleep. Neuroscience. 2002;111(2):231-9. PMID: 11983310.

[804] Bent S, Padula A, Moore D, Patterson M, Mehling W: Valerian for sleep: a systematic review and meta-analysis. 2006. In: Database of Abstracts of Reviews of Effects (DARE): Quality-assessed Reviews [Internet]. York (UK): Centre for Reviews and Dissemination (UK); 1995-2006. Available from: www.ncbi.nlm.nih.gov/books/NBK73156.

[805] Nunes A, Sousa M: Use of valerian in anxiety and sleep disorders: what is the best evidence? Acta Med Port. 2011 Dec;24 Suppl 4:961-6. PMID: 22863505.

[806] Kelber O, Nieber K, Kraft K. Valerian: no evidence for clinically relevant interactions. Evid Based Complement Alternat Med. 2014;2014:879396. doi:10.1155/2014/879396.

[807] Singh O, Khanam Z, Misra N, Srivastava MK. Chamomile (Matricaria chamomilla L.): An overview. Pharmacogn Rev. 2011;5(9):82-95. doi: 10.4103/0973-7847.79103.

[808] Sándor Z, Mottaghipisheh J, Veres K, et al. Evidence Supports Tradition: The in Vitro Effects of Roman Chamomile on Smooth Muscles. Front Pharmacol. 2018;9:323. doi:10.3389/fphar.2018.00323.

[809] Sándor Z, Mottaghipisheh J, Veres K, et al. Evidence Supports Tradition: The in Vitro Effects of Roman Chamomile on Smooth Muscles. Front Pharmacol. 2018;9:323. doi:10.3389/fphar.2018.00323.

[810] Zeggwagh NA, Moufid A, Michel JB, Eddouks M: Hypotensive effect of Chamaemelum nobile aqueous extract in spontaneously hypertensive rats. Clin Exp Hypertens. 2009 Jul;31(5):440-50. PMID: 19811353.

[811] European Health Agency. Assessment Report on Chamaemelum nobile. EMA/HMPC/560906/2010.

[812] Forster HB, Niklas H, Lutz S: Antispasmodic effects of some medicinal plants. Planta Med. 1980 Dec;40(4):309-19. doi: 10.1055/s-2008-1074977.

[813] Adib-Hajbaghery M, Mousavi SN: The effects of chamomile extract on sleep quality among elderly people: A clinical trial. Complement Ther Med. 2017 Dec;35:109-114. doi: 10.1016/j.ctim.2017.09.010.

[814] Kong Y, Wang T, Wang R, Ma Y, Song S, Liu J, Hu W, Li S: Inhalation of Roman chamomile essential oil attenuates depressive-like behaviors in Wistar Kyoto rats. Sci China Life Sci. 2017 Jun;60(6):647-655. doi: 10.1007/s11427-016-9034-8.

[815] Cho MY, Min ES, Hur MH, Lee MS. Effects of aromatherapy on the anxiety, vital signs, and sleep quality of percutaneous coronary intervention patients in intensive care units. Evid Based Complement Alternat Med. 2013;2013:381381. doi:10.1155/2013/381381.

[816] Steward D; The Chemistry of Essential Oils. Care Publications 2013, 4th edition: Chamaemelum nobile. Pg 516-517.

[817] Cortés-Rojas DF, de Souza CR, Oliveira WP. Clove (Syzygium aromaticum): a precious spice. Asian Pac J Trop Biomed. 2014;4(2):90–96. doi:10.1016/S2221-1691(14)60215-X.

[818] Chaieb K, Zmantar T, Ksouri R, Hajlaoui H, Mahdouani K, Abdelly C, Bakhrouf A: Antioxidant properties of the essential oil of Eugenia caryophyllata and its antifungal activity against a large number of clinical Candida species. Mycoses. 2007 Sep;50(5):403-6. doi: 10.1111/j.1439-0507.2007.01391.x.

[819] Gülçin I, Elmastaş M, Aboul-Enein HY. Antioxidant activity of clove oil-A powerful antioxidant source. Arab J Chem. 2012;5(4):489–499. doi.org/10.1016/j.arabjc.2010.09.016.

[820] Nuñez L, Aquino MD. Microbicide activity of clove essential oil (Eugenia caryophyllata). Braz J Microbiol. 2012;43(4):1255–1260. doi:10.1590/S1517-83822012000400003.

[821] Kouidhi B, Zmantar T, Bakhrouf A: Anticariogenic and cytotoxic activity of clove essential oil (Eugenia caryophyllata) against a large number of oral pathogens. Ann Microbiol. 2010;60:599–604.

[822] Chakraborty SK. Halitosis And Mouthwashes. Med J Armed Forces India. 2017;54(3):289–290. doi:10.1016/S0377-1237(17)30576-2.

[823] Mehta AK, Halder S, Khanna N, Tandon OP, Sharma KK: The effect of the essential oil of Eugenia caryophyllata in animal models of depression and

locomotor activity. Nutr Neurosci. 2013 Sep;16(5):233-8. doi: 10.1179/1476830512Y.0000000051.

[824] Halder S, Mehta AK, Kar R, Mustafa M, Mediratta PK, Sharma KK: Clove oil reverses learning and memory deficits in scopolamine-treated mice. Planta Med. 2011 May;77(8):830-4. doi: 10.1055/s-0030-1250605.

[825] Han X, Parker TL. Anti-inflammatory activity of clove (Eugenia caryophyllata) essential oil in human dermal fibroblasts. Pharm Biol. 2017;55(1):1619–1622. doi:10.1080/13880209.2017.1314513.

[826] Halder S, Mehta AK, Mediratta PK, Sharma KK: Acute effect of essential oil of Eugenia caryophyllata on cognition and pain in mice. Naunyn Schmiedebergs Arch Pharmacol. 2012 Jun;385(6):587-93. doi: 10.1007/s00210-012-0742-2.

[827] Kamkar Asl M, Nazariborun A, Hosseini M. Analgesic effect of the aqueous and ethanolic extracts of clove. Avicenna J Phytomed. 2013;3(2):186–192. PMID: 25050273.

[828] Kamkar Asl M, Nazariborun A, Hosseini M. Analgesic effect of the aqueous and ethanolic extracts of clove. Avicenna J Phytomed. 2013;3(2):186–192. PMID: 25050273.

[829] Steward D; The Chemistry of Essential Oils. Care Publications 2013, 4th edition: Syzygium aromatica. Pg 551.

[830] Fine PG, Rosenfeld MJ. The endocannabinoid system, cannabinoids, and pain. Rambam Maimonides Med J. 2013;4(4):e0022. doi:10.5041/RMMJ.10129.

[831] Selim SA, Adam ME, Hassan SM, Albalawi AR. Chemical composition, antimicrobial and antibiofilm activity of the essential oil and methanol extract of the Mediterranean cypress (Cupressus sempervirens L.). BMC Complement Altern Med. 2014;14:179. doi:10.1186/1472-6882-14-179.

[832] Russo EB. Taming THC: potential cannabis synergy and phytocannabinoid-terpenoid entourage effects. Br J Pharmacol. 2011;163(7):1344-64. doi: 10.1111/j.1476-5381.2011.01238.x.

[833] Ibrahim TA, El-Hela AA, El-Hefnawy HM, Al-Taweel AM, Perveen S: Chemical Composition and Antimicrobial Activities of Essential Oils of Some Coniferous Plants Cultivated in Egypt. ran J Pharm Res. 2017 Winter;16(1):328-337. PMID: 28496486.

[834] Lee SH, Do HS, Min KJ. Effects of Essential Oil from Hinoki Cypress, Chamaecyparis obtusa, on Physiology and Behavior of Flies. PLoS One. 2015;10(12):e0143450.. doi:10.1371/journal.pone.0143450.

[835] Raha S, Kim SM, Lee HJ, Lee SJ, Heo JD, Venkatarame Gowda Saralamma V, Ha SE, Kim EH, Mun SP, Kim GS: Essential oil from Korean Chamaecyparis obtusa leaf ameliorates respiratory activity in Sprague-Dawley rats and exhibits protection from NF-κB-induced inflammation in WI38 fibroblast cells. Int J Mol Med. 2019 Jan;43(1):393-403. doi: 10.3892/ijmm.2018.3966. .

[836] Yeşilada E, Sezik E, Honda G, Takaishi Y, Takeda Y, Tanaka T: Traditional medicine in Turkey IX: folk medicine in north-west Anatolia. J Ethnopharmacol. 1999 Mar;64(3):195-210. PMID: 10363834.

[837] Ikei H, Song C, Miyazaki Y: Physiological effect of olfactory stimulation by Hinoki cypress (Chamaecyparis obtusa) leaf oil. J Physiol Anthropol. 2015 Dec 22;34:44. doi: 10.1186/s40101-015-0082-2.

838 Ikei H, Song C, Miyazaki Y: Physiological Effects of Touching the Wood of Hinoki Cypress (Chamaecyparis obtusa) with the Soles of the Feet. Int J Environ Res Public Health. 2018 Sep 28;15(10). pii: E2135. doi: 10.3390/ijerph15102135..

839 Asgary S, Naderi GA, Ardekani MRS, Sahebkar A, Airin A, Aslani S, KasherT, Emami SA: Chemical analysis and biological activities of Cupressus sempervirens var. horizontalis essential oils, Pharmaceutical Biology, (2013) 51:2, 137-144, doi: 10.3109/13880209.2012.715168.

840 Gkogkolou P, Böhm M. Advanced glycation end products: Key players in skin aging?. Dermatoendocrinol. 2012;4(3):259-70..

841 Moy RL, Levenson C. Sandalwood Album Oil as a Botanical Therapeutic in Dermatology. J Clin Aesthet Dermatol. 2017;10(10):34-39. PMID: 29344319.

842 Sharma M, Levenson C, Browning JC, Becker EM, Clements I, Castella P, Cox ME: East Indian Sandalwood Oil Is a Phosphodiesterase Inhibitor: A New Therapeutic Option in the Treatment of Inflammatory Skin Disease. Front Pharmacol. 2018 Mar 9;9:200. doi: 10.3389/fphar.2018.00200.

843 Warnke PH, Becker ST, Podschun R, Sivananthan S, Springer IN, Russo PA, Wiltfang J, Fickenscher H, Sherry E: The battle against multi-resistant strains: Renaissance of antimicrobial essential oils as a promising force to fight hospital-acquired infections. J Craniomaxillofac Surg. 2009 Oct;37(7):392-7. doi: 10.1016/j.jcms.2009.03.017.

844 Gupta PD, Birdi TJ: Development of botanicals to combat antibiotic resistance. J Ayurveda Integr Med. 2017 Oct - Dec;8(4):266-275. doi: 10.1016/j.jaim.2017.05.004.

845 Santha S, Dwivedi C: Anticancer Effects of Sandalwood (Santalum album). Anticancer Res. 2015 Jun;35(6):3137-45. PMID: 26026073.

846 Dwivedi C, Guan X, Harmsen WL, Voss AL, Goetz-Parten DE, Koopman EM, Johnson KM, Valluri HB, Matthees DP: Chemopreventive effects of alpha-santalol on skin tumor development in CD-1 and SENCAR mice. Cancer Epidemiol Biomarkers Prev. 2003 Feb;12(2):151-6. PMID: 12582025.

847 Dwivedi C, Zhang Y: Sandalwood oil prevent skin tumour development in CD1 mice. Eur J Cancer Prev. 1999 Oct;8(5):449-55. PMID: 10548401.

848 Zhang X, Dwivedi C: Skin cancer chemoprevention by α-santalol. Front Biosci (Schol Ed). 2011 Jan 1;3:777-87. PMID: 21196411.

849 Dwivedi C, Valluri HB, Guan X, Agarwal R: Chemopreventive effects of alpha-santalol on ultraviolet B radiation-induced skin tumor development in SKH-1 hairless mice. Carcinogenesis. 2006 Sep;27(9):1917-22. doi: 10.1093/carcin/bgl058.

850 Bommareddy A, Hora J, Cornish B, Dwivedi C: Chemoprevention by alpha-santalol on UVB radiation-induced skin tumor development in mice. Anticancer Res. 2007 Jul-Aug;27(4B):2185-8. PMID: 17695502.

851 Dozmorov MG, Yang Q, Wu W, et al. Differential effects of selective frankincense (Ru Xiang) essential oil versus non-selective sandalwood (Tan Xiang) essential oil on cultured bladder cancer cells: a microarray and bioinformatics study. Chin Med. 2014;9:18. doi:10.1186/1749-8546-9-18.

852 Lee B, Bohmann J, Reeves T, Levenson C, Risinger AL: α- and β-Santalols Directly Interact with Tubulin and Cause Mitotic Arrest and Cytotoxicity in

Oral Cancer Cells. J Nat Prod. 2015 Jun 26;78(6):1357-62. doi: 10.1021/acs.jnatprod.5b00207.

[853] Denda M: Newly discovered olfactory receptors in epidermal keratinocytes are associated with proliferation, migration, and re-epithelialization of keratinocytes. J Invest Dermatol. 2014 Nov;134(11):2677-2679. doi: 10.1038/jid.2014.229.

[854] Oh SJ. System-Wide Expression and Function of Olfactory Receptors in Mammals. Genomics Inform. 2018;16(1):2-9. doi: 10.5808/GI.2018.16.1.2.

[855] Busse D, Kudella P, Grüning NM, Gisselmann G, Ständer S, Luger T, Jacobsen F, Steinsträßer L, Paus R, Gkogkolou P, Böhm M, Hatt H, Benecke H: A synthetic sandalwood odorant induces wound-healing processes in human keratinocytes via the olfactory receptor OR2AT4. J Invest Dermatol. 2014 Nov;134(11):2823-2832. doi: 10.1038/jid.2014.273.

[856] Chéret J, Bertolini M, Ponce L, Lehmann J, Tsai T, Alam M, Hatt H, Paus R: Olfactory receptor OR2AT4 regulates human hair growth. Nat Commun. 2018 Sep 18;9(1):3624. doi: 10.1038/s41467-018-05973-0.

[857] Weber L, Maßberg D, Becker C, et al. Olfactory Receptors as Biomarkers in Human Breast Carcinoma Tissues. Front Oncol. 2018;8:33. doi:10.3389/fonc.2018.00033.

[858] Antunes Viegas D, Palmeira-de-Oliveira A, Salgueiro L, Martinez-de-Oliveira J, Palmeira-de-Oliveira R: Helichrysum italicum: from traditional use to scientific data. J Ethnopharmacol. 2014;151(1):54-65. doi: 10.1016/j.jep.2013.11.005.

[859] Appendino G, Gibbons S, Giana A, Pagani A, Grassi G, Stavri M, Smith E, Rahman MM: Antibacterial cannabinoids from Cannabis sativa: a structure-activity study. J Nat Prod. 2008 Aug;71(8):1427-30. doi: 10.1021/np8002673.

[860] Andre CM, Hausman JF, Guerriero G. Cannabis sativa: The Plant of the Thousand and One Molecules. Front Plant Sci. 2016;7:19. doi:10.3389/fpls.2016.00019.

[861] Bohlmann F, Hoffmann E. Cannabigerol-ähnliche verbindungen aus Helichrysum umbraculigerum. Phytochemistry 1979;18:1371–4.

[862] Djihane B, Wafa N, Elkhamssa S, Pedro HJ, Maria AE, Mohamed Mihoub Z. Chemical constituents of Helichrysum italicum (Roth) G. Don essential oil and their antimicrobial activity against Gram-positive and Gram-negative bacteria, filamentous fungi and Candida albicans. Saudi Pharm J. 2016;25(5):780-787. doi: 10.1016/j.jsps.2016.11.001.

[863] Antunes Viegas D, Palmeira-de-Oliveira A, Salgueiro L, Martinez-de-Oliveira J, Palmeira-de-Oliveira R: Helichrysum italicum: from traditional use to scientific data. J Ethnopharmacol. 2014;151(1):54-65. doi: 10.1016/j.jep.2013.11.005.

[864] Sala A, Recio M, Giner RM, Máñez S, Tournier H, Schinella G, Ríos JL: Anti-inflammatory and antioxidant properties of Helichrysum italicum. J Pharm Pharmacol. 2002 Mar;54(3):365-71. PMID: 11902802.

[865] Süntar I, Küpeli Akkol E, Keles H, Yesilada E, Sarker SD: Exploration of the wound healing potential of Helichrysum graveolens (Bieb.) Sweet: isolation of apigenin as an active component. J Ethnopharmacol. 2013 Aug 26;149(1):103-10. doi: 10.1016/j.jep.2013.06.006.

[866] Stewart D: The Chemistry of Essential Oils Made Simple. Chemical Analysis of Helichrysum. Care Publications 2013. Pg 531.

[867] Hanuš LO, Meyer SM, Muñoz E, Taglialatela-Scafati), Appendino G: Phytocannabinoids: a unified critical inventory. Nat. Prod. Rep., 2016, 33, 1357-1392. doi: 10.1039/C6NP00074F.

[868] Stewart D: The Chemistry of Essential Oils Made Simple. Chemical Analysis of Piper Nigrum. Care Publications 2013. Table 32. P 545..

[869] Han X, Beaumont C, Rodriguez D, Bahr T: Black pepper (Piper nigrum) essential oil demonstrates tissue remodeling and metabolism modulating potential in human cells. Phytother Res. 2018 Sep;32(9):1848-1852. doi: 10.1002/ptr.6110..

[870] Vinturelle R, Mattos C, Meloni J, et al. In Vitro Evaluation of Essential Oils Derived from Piper nigrum (Piperaceae) and Citrus limonum (Rutaceae) against the Tick Rhipicephalus (Boophilus) microplus (Acari: Ixodidae). Biochem Res Int. 2017;2017:5342947. doi: 10.1155/2017/5342947.

[871] Kapoor IP, Singh B, Singh G, De Heluani CS, De Lampasona MP, Catalan CA: Chemistry and in vitro antioxidant activity of volatile oil and oleoresins of black pepper (Piper nigrum). J Agric Food Chem. 2009 Jun 24;57(12):5358-64. doi: 10.1021/jf900642x.

[872] Bagheri H, Abdul Manap MY, Solati Z: Antioxidant activity of Piper nigrum L. essential oil extracted by supercritical CO_2 extraction and hydro-distillation. Talanta. 2014 Apr;121:220-8. doi: 10.1016/j.talanta.2014.01.007.

[873] Butt MS, Pasha I, Sultan MT, Randhawa MA, Saeed F, Ahmed W: Black pepper and health claims: a comprehensive treatise. Crit Rev Food Sci Nutr. 2013;53(9):875-86. doi: 10.1080/10408398.2011.571799.

[874] Ou MC, Lee YF, Li CC, Wu SK: The effectiveness of essential oils for patients with neck pain: a randomized controlled study. J Altern Complement Med. 2014 Oct;20(10):771-9. doi: 10.1089/acm.2013.0453.

[875] Kristiniak S, Harpel J, Breckenridge DM, Buckle J: Black pepper essential oil to enhance intravenous catheter insertion in patients with poor vein visibility: a controlled study. J Altern Complement Med. 2012 Nov;18(11):1003-7. doi: 10.1089/acm.2012.0106.

[876] Cherniakov I, Izgelov D, Barasch D, Davidson E, Domb AJ, Hoffman A: Piperine-pro-nanolipospheres as a novel oral delivery system of cannabinoids: Pharmacokinetic evaluation in healthy volunteers in comparison to buccal spray administration. J Control Release. 2017 Nov 28;266:1-7. doi: 10.1016/j.jconrel.2017.09.011.

[877] Cherniakov I, Izgelov D, Domb AJ, Hoffman A: The effect of Pro NanoLipospheres (PNL) formulation containing natural absorption enhancers on the oral bioavailability of delta-9-tetrahydrocannabinol (THC) and cannabidiol (CBD) in a rat model. Eur J Pharm Sci. 2017 Nov 15;109:21-30. doi: 10.1016/j.ejps.2017.07.003.

[878] Steward D; The Chemistry of Essential Oils. Care Publications 2013, 4th edition: Salvia officinalis. Pg 548.

[879] Olson R: Absinthe and γ-aminobutyric acid receptors. Proceedings of the National Academy of Sciences Apr 2000, 97 (9) 4417-4418; doi: 10.1073/pnas.97.9.4417.

[880] Albert-Puleo M: Van Gogh's vision: thujone intoxication. JAMA. 1981 Jul 3;246(1):42. PMID: 7017175.

[881] Arnold WN: Vincent van Gogh and the thujone connection. JAMA. 1988 Nov 25;260(20):3042-4. PMID: 3054185.

[882] Arnold WN, Loftus LS: Xanthopsia and van Gogh's yellow palette. Eye (Lond). 1991;5 (Pt 5):503-10. doi: 10.1038/eye.1991.93.

[883] Lachenmeier DW, Emmert J, Kuballa T, Sartor G: Thujone--cause of absinthism? Forensic Sci Int. 2006 Apr 20;158(1):1-8. doi: 10.1016/j.forsciint.2005.04.010.

[884] Höld KM, Sirisoma NS, Ikeda T, Narahashi T, Casida JE. Alpha-thujone (the active component of absinthe): gamma-aminobutyric acid type A receptor modulation and metabolic detoxification. Proc Natl Acad Sci U S A. 2000;97(8):3826-31. doi: 10.1073/pnas.070042397.

[885] Meschler JP, Howlett AC: Thujone exhibits low affinity for cannabinoid receptors but fails to evoke cannabimimetic responses. Pharmacol Biochem Behav. 1999 Mar;62(3):473-80. PMID: 10080239.

[886] Medicinal Plants: Medicinal Plants Modulating Cannabinoid Receptors and Endocannabinoid Metabolizing Enzymes. Phytochemistry, Pharmacology and Therapeutics, Edition: 4, Chapter: 13, Publisher: Daya Publishing House®, Editors: V.K. Gupta, G.D. Singh, Surjeet Singh, A. Kaul, pp.285-302.

[887] Sharma C, Sadek B, Goyal SN, Sinha S, Kamal MA, Ojha S: Small Molecules from Nature Targeting G-Protein Coupled Cannabinoid Receptors: Potential Leads for Drug Discovery and Development. Evidence-Based Complementary and Alternative Medicine. Volume 2015, Article ID 238482, 26 pages. doi.org/10.1155/2015/238482.

[888] Zgair A, Wong JC, Lee JB, et al. Dietary fats and pharmaceutical lipid excipients increase systemic exposure to orally administered cannabis and cannabis-based medicines. Am J Transl Res. 2016;8(8):3448–3459. Published 2016 Aug 15.

[889] Zgair A, Lee JB, Wong JCM, Taha DA, Aram J, Di Virgilio D, McArthur JW, Cheng YK, Hennig IM, Barrett DA, Fischer PM, Constantinescu CS, Gershkovich P: Oral administration of cannabis with lipids leads to high levels of cannabinoids in the intestinal lymphatic system and prominent immunomodulation. Sci Rep. 2017 Nov 6;7(1):14542. doi: 10.1038/s41598-017-15026-z.

[890] Cherniakov I, Izgelov D, Domb AJ, Hoffman A: The effect of Pro NanoLipospheres (PNL) formulation containing natural absorption enhancers on the oral bioavailability of delta-9-tetrahydrocannabinol (THC) and cannabidiol (CBD) in a rat model. Eur J Pharm Sci. 2017 Nov 15;109:21-30. doi: 10.1016/j.ejps.2017.07.003.

[891] Zitter JN, Mazonson PD, Miller DP, Hulley SB, Balmes JR: Aircraft cabin air recirculation and symptoms of the common cold. JAMA. 2002 Jul 24-31;288(4):483-6. PMID: 12132979.

[892] Moser MR, Bender TR, Margolis HS, Noble GR, Kendal AP, Ritter DG: An outbreak of influenza aboard a commercial airliner. Am J Epidemiol. 1979 Jul;110(1):1-6. PMID: 463858.